ATLAS of POST-MORTEM TECHNIQUES
in NEUROPATHOLOGY

ATLAS of POST-MORTEM TECHNIQUES
in NEUROPATHOLOGY

J. HUME ADAMS
Professor of Neuropathology
University Department of Neuropathology
Institute of Neurological Sciences,
Southern General Hospital,
Glasgow, Scotland

and

MARGARET F. MURRAY
Senior Medical Photographer
Regional Plastic and Oral Surgery Unit
Canniesburn Hospital
Glasgow, Scotland

CAMBRIDGE UNIVERSITY PRESS
Cambridge
London   New York   New Rochelle
Melbourne   Sydney

CAMBRIDGE UNIVERSITY PRESS
Cambridge, New York, Melbourne, Madrid, Cape Town, Singapore, São Paulo, Delhi

Cambridge University Press
The Edinburgh Building, Cambridge CB2 8RU, UK

Published in the United States of America by Cambridge University Press, New York

www.cambridge.org
Information on this title: www.cambridge.org/9780521105682

First published 1982
This digitally printed version 2009

A catalogue record for this publication is available from the British Library

Library of Congress Catalogue Card Number: 82–4313

ISBN 978-0-521-24121-2 hardback
ISBN 978-0-521-10568-2 paperback

Contents

Foreword   vii

Preface   ix

1. The Brain   1

2. The Base of the Skull   34

3. The Eye and Orbital Contents   44

4. The Spinal Cord   67

5. The Extracranial Cerebral Arteries
   in the Neck   82

6. Muscle and Nerve   91

7. Dissection of the Fixed Brain   96

8. The Anatomy of the Brain   116

Foreword

There is no doubt that the ever-increasing number
and variety of investigations applicable during life has
led to considerable improvements in diagnostic practice,
and in consequence there is now a tendency to downgrade
the clinical importance of the autopsy.   This is
unfortunate, for every competent pathologist knows that,
quite apart from its teaching value, autopsy commonly
reveals lesions which, had they been appreciated earlier,
would have influenced the management of the patient
concerned.   Indeed, this has been confirmed by recent
collaborative studies between pathologists and clinicians
practicing a high standard of patient care.   Yet even
the most conscientious pathologist may have difficulty
in providing an adequate autopsy service, for the
diagnostic biopsy service must claim first priority, and
this has increased greatly as a result of advances in
radiological and related procedures, in endoscopy and
in needle biopsy techniques.
    If the autopsy is to hold its place as a helpful
investigative procedure and a means of medical audit, it
is essential that it should be performed in such a way
as to provide the greatest amount of useful information,
and nowhere is technique more important than in the
removal and preservation of the tissues dealt with in
this book - the nervous and muscular systems and the eye.
Unlike his clinical contemporaries, who have undergone a
fair apprenticeship in the major bedside specialties
during the medical school curriculum and early post-

graduate training, the trainee pathologist has usually
little or no previous practical experience in his
intended specialty. He (or she) will find this book
invaluable, for although atlases and texts on general
autopsy technique are available, I know of none which
deals with these topics as clearly and authoritatively
as in the pages which follow. Nor are Professor Adams
and his colleagues alone among neuropathologists in
lamenting the uneven standard of autopsy practice,
sometimes even by experienced pathologists, in this
country. To the consultant pathologist, the advice
they offer will not only improve the value of autopsies,
but will actually save time by excluding many of the
artefacts which arise from unsatisfactory technique and
which render diagnosis more difficult.

Finally, it seems appropriate to note that the
Neuropathology Department in the West of Scotland, which
was instituted by my predecessor, Professor D.F. Cappell,
has for many years provided a superb referral service
to pathologists in the region. I hope that we can now
express our appreciation by improving the quality of
material submitted to Professor Adams and his colleagues.

                                        J.R. Anderson

University Department of Pathology,
Western Infirmary,
Glasgow.

Preface

    As every neuropathologist knows, the brain and
spinal cord are often not removed as well as they
should be post mortem: it is very frustrating to be
asked to undertake a neuropathological assessment on
specimens that are so distorted that it is difficult, if
not impossible, to reconstitute the situation that
existed prior to death. Yet this is precisely the information sought by neurosurgeon, neurologist and neuro-
radiologist. Since it is not difficult to remove the
brain and cord properly, one can only assume that
pathologists and mortuary attendants are unaware of the
importance of doing so. A common reason for a brain
becoming distorted is that it is removed by the mortuary
attendant and then left lying on the dissecting bench
for some time before the pathologist decides that it
should be fixed intact for dissection later. Furthermore, the optic chiasma and the brain stem are often
torn, and the lower medulla and the vertebral arteries
are often left within the skull. These observations
are not meant to be critical of mortuary attendants,
but more of pathologists who fail to appreciate the
importance of removing the brain themselves, or at least
being present when it is being removed. How else can
they know if the dura is tight or slack, and if there is
any blood in the extradural or subdural spaces, or how
much blood, or for that matter in what space!
    This book is therefore aimed at general pathologists
and mortuary attendants in the hope of convincing them

that it is not difficult or time-consuming to remove
and fix the brain and spinal cord properly post mortem.
Neuropathology is simply a branch of general pathology
and we would hope to persuade general pathologists to
take a more active interest in the brain and to dissect
brains themselves after fixation.   So much more information becomes available to clinician and pathologist
if the brain is properly fixed and dissected that it is
difficult ever to justify slicing at the time of autopsy
the brain of a patient dying as a result of some neurological disorder.

Some time ago we were invited by the World Health
Organization, as part of their UND/World Bank/WHO
Special Programme for Research and Training in Tropical
Diseases, to produce an illustrated manual on how to
remove the brain.   This was to be used by medical
practitioners in various African countries, often in
poorly equipped hospitals away from major medical
centres, on patients dying as a result of African
trypanosomiasis.   Since the brains we have received
from these sources have often been in much better con-
dition than those we receive from Departments of Pathology in the West of Scotland, it occurred to us and
Cambridge University Press that a similar manual might
be of more general interest.   We are greatly indebted
to the WHO Special Programme for allowing us to re-
produce in this atlas several of the original illustrations, viz. Figs. 1.1-1.3, 1.11-1.26, 1.28-1.30,
1.33 and 2.2-2.6.

We have, however, incorporated several new features
viz. how to remove the spinal cord and posterior root
ganglia, how to examine the base of the skull, how to
dissect out the major extracranial cerebral arteries in
the neck and how to take samples of nerve and muscle.
We are particularly indebted to Professor W.R. Lee,

Professor of Ophthalmic Pathology in the University of
Glasgow, for collaborating with Mrs. Murray in the
preparation of chapter 3 which deals with the eye and
orbital contents.   And finally, in the hope of per-
suading more pathologists to fix and dissect brains,
there are chapters on how to dissect a fixed brain and
on neuro-anatomy.   The last chapter is not meant to
compete with comprehensive textbooks of neuro-anatomy
but it is hoped that it will help pathologists to de-
lineate reasonably precisely the anatomical distribution
of any structural abnormalities they observe in the
brain.

In countries where embalming is practised widely,
some of the techniques described may require to be
modified but none is incompatible with proper re-
constitution of the body.   The general principles
remain: good exposure, careful removal and proper
fixation.

We have already expressed our appreciation of the
invaluable help given to us by Professor W.R. Lee.   We
would also like to thank Mrs. Joan Rubython for her
tireless and uncomplaining secretarial assistance: we
are now very conscious of the work entailed in producing camera-ready copy.   We are also greatly indebted to Professor J.R. Anderson for his Foreword,
and to Cambridge University Press for their courteous
and helpful approach to all our queries and, in
particular, to the generous assistance given to us by
Mr. Jack Bowles and Dr. Fay Bendall.

J. Hume Adams

Glasgow   Margaret F. Murray

1. The Brain

Before commencing a post-mortem examination on any patient known to have had some neurological disease, the pathologist must consider - preferably in consultation with the clinician - what special steps might have to be undertaken prior to fixing the brain. If there is any clinical suspicion of meningitis, some of the exudate should be sent for bacteriological examination - micro-biologists prefer exudate itself rather than a swab; if any type of encephalitis has been considered in the differential diagnosis, representative samples of brain tissue should be placed in an appropriate transport medium and sent for virological examination - and also samples of blood and cerebrospinal fluid for serological studies; if there is a possibility of some lysosomal enzyme deficiency, e.g. one of the neuronal storage disorders, or an unusual type of demyelinating disease, some brain tissue should be deep frozen as quickly as possible in case it is required later for neurochemical analysis; and if the post-mortem examination is being undertaken soon after death, the possibility of taking samples of the brain for electron microscopy should be borne in mind.

There are two basic principles in removing the brain - all structures holding it in position must be cut without inflicting any damage on the brain, and un-due stretching of the brain stem must be avoided since it is very liable to tear at the level of the midbrain (see Fig. 1.26). It is not difficult to remove a

normal brain if an adequate exposure has been attained.
If, however, it is enlarged for any reason, either as a
result of an intracranial expanding lesion or of diffuse
brain swelling, the increased volume of the brain makes
access to the various structures that have to be cut
more difficult.   In such circumstances, therefore,
particular care has to be exercised.   Furthermore, if
there is blood or pus in the subarachnoid space, many
of the structures to be cut are obscured and sometimes
some of these have to be cut blind.   Hence the
importance of becoming competent in removing normal
brains so that one already knows the technique.

    Before starting to remove the brain examine the
scalp, face and neck carefully for any lacerations,
abrasions or surgical incisions.   Pay particular
attention to the occipital region since lesions there
are often not immediately obvious.   Retract the eyelids to see if there is any subconjunctival haemorrhage.

    Figs. 1.1 and 1.2 Make a transverse incision with
a scalpel through the scalp, starting behind one ear
and ending behind the other.

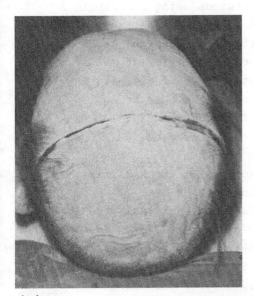

1.1

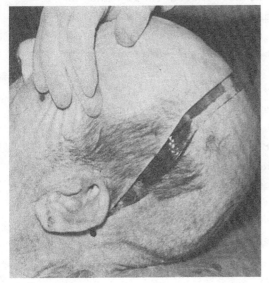

1.2

Fig. 1.3   Reflect the scalp forwards using a scalpel
where required to separate the scalp from the skull up
to but not beyond the supra-orbital ridges (the level of
the eyebrows).   Reflect the scalp in a similar manner
posteriorly towards the occiput.   Note if there is any
blood clot deep to the scalp and if there is any
haemorrhage into or bruising of its deep surface.   Examine the vault of the skull for any evidence of
fracture and note its size and its location.   One of
the best ways of recording fractures of the skull is
diagrammatically on line drawings of the skull.   Note
also the size and position of any neurosurgical procedures, such as burr holes or a craniotomy.

   Removal of too small a portion of the vault of the
skull is one of the commonest faults in neuropathological post-mortem technique: a large part has to be
taken away if the brain is to be removed easily and un-
damaged.   Anteriorly the saw cut should lie about 1.0
cm above the supra-orbital ridge and then be continued
horizontally on each side to behind the ear.

Fig. 1.4   As a preliminary step it is helpful to cut
through the temporal muscle at this level and scrape
some of it off the skull for a short distance above and
below this incision so that the saw will have clear
access to the bone.   If the cut in the temporal muscle
is made lower than suggested, the saw will go through
the petrous part of the temporal bone leaving a sharp
bony spur on the skull cap which will inevitably damage
the brain when the skull cap is being removed.

5

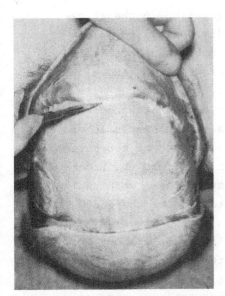

1.3

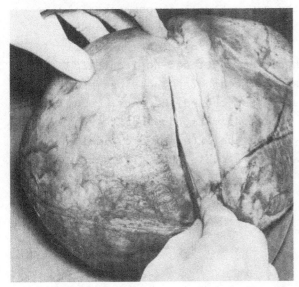

1.4

Figs. 1.5 - 1.7 There is great variation in the thickness of the skull in different individuals, and in any
individual it is thicker in the frontal and occipital
regions than in the temporal bone immediately above the
ear. Since it is important to try to leave the dura -
the fibrous sheet immediately deep to and attached to
the skull - intact, the undersurface of the spindle of
the saw should be supported by one hand so as to prevent
the saw blade plunging through the dura into the underlying brain. Particular care must be taken when sawing
through the temporal bone immediately above the ear
since the bone here is often as thin as 2-3 mm.
    The saw cut should be started anteriorly about 1 cm
above the level of the supra-orbital ridges. If the
cut is made higher than this, difficulty will be en-
countered later in freeing the frontal lobes. If it is
made lower than this, the saw cut will almost certainly
go through the frontal sinuses; this, however, is not
a very serious problem unless the sinuses are unusually
large. The saw cut should be continued horizontally
on either side of the skull through the incisions made
in the temporal muscles to just behind the ears. The
saw cut should then be angled slightly upwards to reach
the midline immediately above the external occipital
protuberance which is easily palpable as a distinct
prominence at the back of the skull.

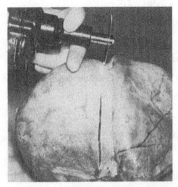

1.5

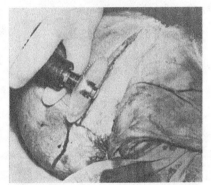

1.6

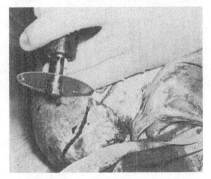

1.7

Figs. 1.8 and 1.9   Prise the skull cap loose by
twisting a T-shaped chisel along the saw cut.   A
gentle tap with a mallet is permissible at this stage if
the skull has not been completely cut through.   Strong
hammering must be avoided since this may produce damage
to the bone that might be misinterpreted as a fracture.
It is essential that the skull cap be loosened around
the entire saw cut before any attempt is made to remove
it.

        Note if any blood or fluid runs out of the skull
as the skull cap is being freed from the remainder of
the skull, and try to measure its approximate volume.

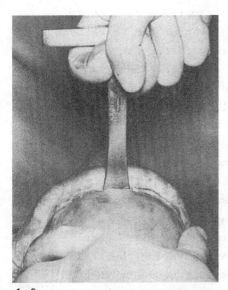

1.8

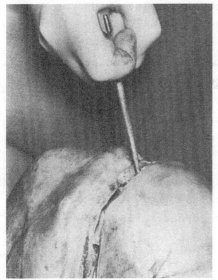

1.9

Figs. 1.10 and 1.11   The dura is sometimes so loosely
attached to the skull cap that the latter can be removed
fairly easily simply by pulling it with the fingers
backwards from the forehead.   On the other hand,
particularly in old age and in infancy, the dura may be
very firmly adherent to the skull cap with the result
that it can only be removed with considerable difficulty.
In these circumstances it is helpful to insert a
malleable spatula (Fig. 1.10) between the dura and the
skull cap to help to separate one from the other.   Care
must be taken not to damage the surface of the brain but
this can usually be avoided if the dura was not opened
when the saw cut was being made in the skull.   When
some difficulty is experienced in separating the skull
cap from the dura, there is a distinct tendency when
retracting the skull cap from the forehead for the
posterior part of the skull cap to plunge into the
occipital lobes.   This can really only be prevented if
virtually complete separation of the dura from the skull
cap has been achieved with the spatula.   If the dura is
particularly adherent, less damage is likely to be done
to the brain if the skull cap is retracted forwards and
upwards from the occipital region.   When the skull cap
has been removed, the underlying dura should be intact
(Fig. 1.11).

Most extradural haematomas tend to remain attached
to the dura and if one is present its site, size and
approximate thickness should be recorded before pro-
ceeding further.

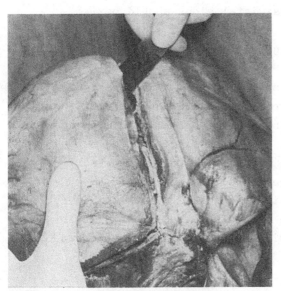

1.10

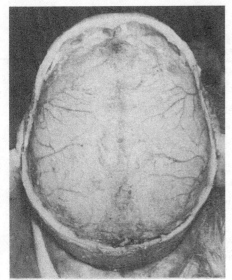

1.11

Fig. 1.12   The superior sagittal sinus should be
opened by incising it posteriorly with a scalpel and
then opening its full length with scissors.

Fig. 1.13   The dura can now be opened.   Seize the dura
with a pair of toothed forceps to one side of the midline in the frontal region and make a small incision at
the level of the saw cut.   Continue incising the dura
along the line of the saw cut using a pair of curved-
on-the-flat scissors since these are less liable to
damage the underlying brain than a scalpel or a bistoury.
The tightness of the dura should be assessed when it is
being incised since this is the only time that this can
be done.

    If the dura is slack and the underlying sub-
arachnoid space contains rather gelatinous cerebrospinal fluid, there is almost certainly some degree of
cerebral atrophy.   If the dura is tight, there is almost certainly an intracranial expanding lesion or
diffuse brain swelling.   The surface of the brain deep
to the dura will be dry and flattened because of ob-
literation of the subarachnoid space.   Since the
surface of the brain will also be in very close contact
with the dura, the dura must be cut in very small bites,
the scissors being kept very close to the forceps
retracting the dura.   If this is not done it is very
easy to damage the surface of the brain with the blunt
edge of the scissors.

    Continue this cut along the saw cut to, but not
cutting through, the superior sagittal sinus.

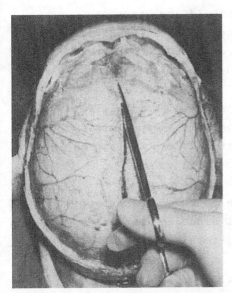

1.12

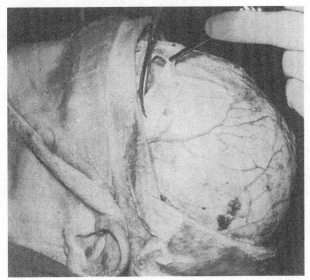

1.13

Fig. 1.14   A similar procedure should now be undertaken to open the dura on the other side of the skull.
The scissors should be turned through 180° so that the
curvature of the blades can be adapted to the shape of
the skull.

Any blood in the subdural space, unless it is an
encapsulated chronic subdural haematoma, tends to flow
out at this stage.   Its colour should be noted and an
attempt made to measure its approximate volume.

Fig. 1.15   Each half of the dura must now be retracted
medially to the superior sagittal sinus, and small
vessels or adhesions cut with scissors.

If any pus or blood is seen on the surface of the
brain when the dura has been retracted, it is in the
subdural space if it can be easily wiped off, but if it
cannot, it lies in the subarachnoid space and is kept in
position by the arachnoid.

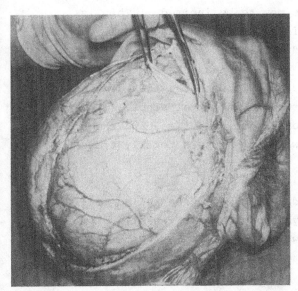

1.14

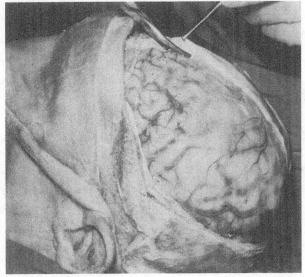

1.15

Fig. 1.16   The falx has now to be incised.   This is
again best done with scissors after pulling gently on
the flaps of dura already reflected from the hemispheres.   The scissors are inserted between the
hemispheres in the frontal region and the falx divided
at right angles to the superior sagittal sinus.   This
should be done in cuts of 2-3 mm at a time, and the falx
will be felt to 'give' when it has been totally transected.

Fig. 1.17   The entire dura should now be pulled gently
backwards.   It normally separates fairly easily from
the brain although a few small vessels (arrows) feeding
into the superior sagittal sinus - bridging veins -
still require to be cut at this stage.

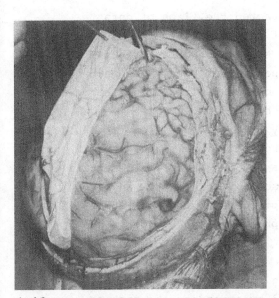

1.16

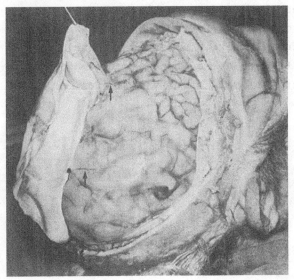

1.17

Fig. 1.18   When fully retracted the flaps of dura
should be left dangling out of the back of the skull.
There is almost invariably some loose dura (arrows)
deep to the remainder of the frontal bone.   As much of
this as possible should be cut away without inflicting
any damage on the adjacent brain.

   The brain is now ready to be removed from the skull.
The most satisfactory instrument to use to cut through
cranial nerves and arteries and the tentorium cerebelli
is curved-on-the-flat scissors.   If properly angled,
the flat surface can be kept close to the bone and the
tearing almost invariably produced by a bistoury or a
scalpel can be avoided.

Fig. 1.19   Before starting to remove the brain, the
head should be repositioned by extending the neck so
that gravity contributes as much as possible to
separating the brain from the base of the skull.   The
fingers should be carefully inserted under the frontal
poles to separate them from the base of the skull and
the olfactory bulbs gently elevated from the base of
the skull.

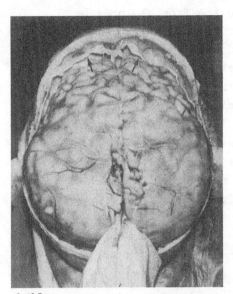

1.18

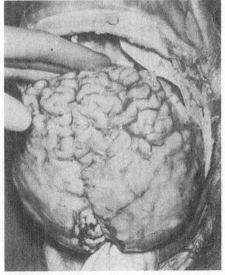

1.19

Fig. 1.20   On no account should the frontal lobes be
pulled away from the base of the skull since this will
almost inevitably tear the optic chiasma and the hypothalamus.   Indeed this is probably the commonest error
made in the course of removing the brain from the skull.
If the head is in the proper position, the frontal lobes
will separate from the anterior fossa as soon as the
olfactory bulbs have been released.   The first major
structures to come into view are the optic nerves
(arrows) and each of these should be cut individually
immediately proximal to the optic foramina.

Fig. 1.21   The internal carotid arteries (arrows) can
then be clearly seen.   These should be cut individually
just where they emerge from the cavernous sinus.

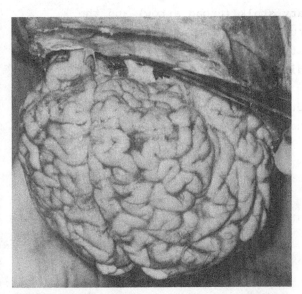

1.20

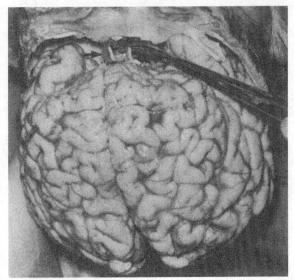

1.21

Fig. 1.22   The pituitary stalk (broad arrow) and the oculomotor nerves (narrow arrows) can now be clearly seen.   The pituitary stalk should now be transected immediately above the diaphragma sellae.

Fig. 1.23   The oculomotor nerves should be cut as close to the base of the skull as possible.

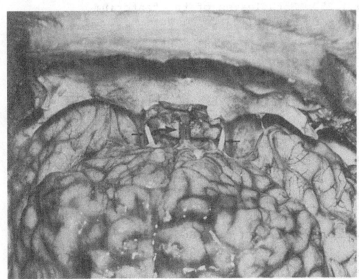

1.22

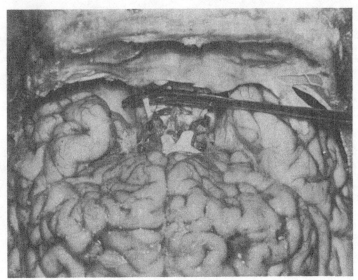

1.23

Figs. 1.24 and 1.25   Both leaves of the tentorium
cerebelli have now to be incised along their attachment
to the petrous parts of the temporal bones.   Gentle
lateral retraction of each hemisphere is required to
achieve this, and this stage in the removal of the brain
may be a little difficult if the brain is swollen.
Using curved scissors in alignment with the petrous part
of the temporal bone, incise the tentorium medially and
then cut along it to the lateral wall of the skull.
Each cut should be of only a few mm in length since it is
very easy to damage the superior surface of the cerebellum with the blunt edge of the scissors.   A similar
incision but with the scissors reversed so that their
flat surface is aligned with the other petrous ridge
should then be undertaken on the other side.

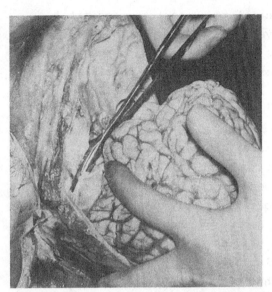

1.24

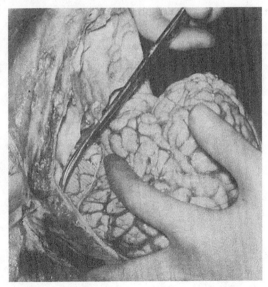

1.25

Fig. 1.26   It is now essential to support the occipital
lobes with one hand to prevent any tearing of the mid-
brain (arrow).   All of the remaining cranial nerves
should be transected as close to the bone as possible.
In the figure opposite the left fifth (trigeminal)
nerve is being cut.

Fig. 1.27   The vertebral arteries have now to be cut.
These must be cut individually since if they are simply
cut through when the upper end of the spinal cord is
being transected, they almost invariably tear with the
result that a considerable amount of each vertebral
artery and indeed even the origins of one or both
posterior inferior cerebellar arteries may remain in
the base of the skull.   Thus each vertebral artery
(arrow) should be transected with curved scissors
immediately above its point of entry into the skull.

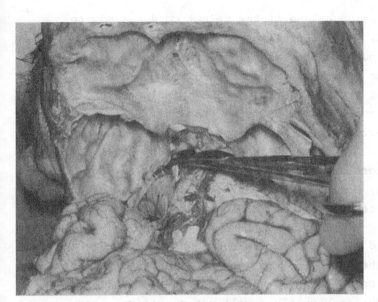

1.26

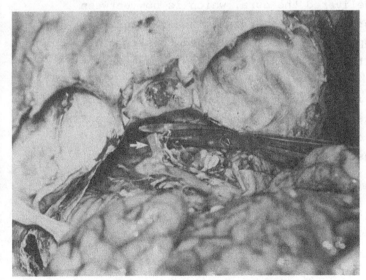

1.27

Fig. 1.28   The upper end of the spinal cord has now to
be transected, preferably with a scalpel.   Only too
often one encounters specimens where there is a
tapering wedge of spinal cord attached to the medulla
as a result of trying to transect the spinal cord as
low down as possible.   This means that the spino-
medullary junction and the upper segments of the spinal
cord cannot be properly examined.   The cervical cord
should therefore be transected transversely (see Fig.
1.31) just at, or above, the cervico-medullary junction.
When it has been completely transected it 'gives'.

Figs. 1.29 and 1.30   The brain can now be delivered
gently from the skull.   It may be necessary to exert
slight traction on the undersurface of the cerebellar
hemispheres but gravity alone will often suffice.   As
the brain is delivered the dura, which is now between
the hand supporting the cerebral hemispheres and the
cerebral hemispheres, should be allowed to slip gently
away so that it still remains attached to the skull.

   If there is a lesion in the lower medulla and/or
in the upper cervical spinal canal, the upper segments
of the spinal cord should be removed attached to the
brain (see Figs. 4.14 to 4.16).

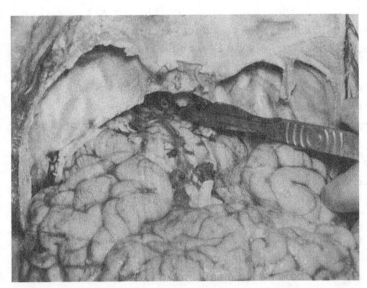

1.28

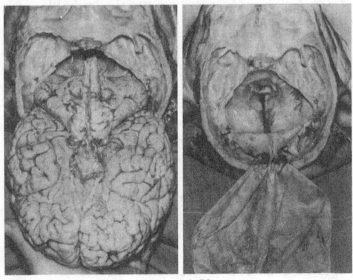

1.29   1.30

Fig. 1.31   This shows the level at which the spinal
cord should be cut transversely.   Note also where the
vertebral arteries enter the skull. (arrows).

Fig. 1.32   The final step in this part of the examination is to strip the dura from the base of the skull
to look for fractures or other bony abnormalities such
as defects in the bone overlying the middle ear or the
mastoid cavity as a result of chronic suppurative
osteitis.   Whether this is done before the special
procedures described in Chapter 2 will depend on the
type of case.   If the principal reason is to look for
a fracture in a fatal head injury, however, the only
procedure that requires to be undertaken before
stripping the dura is to incise the posterior margin of
the diaphragma sellae (Fig. 2.2).   To strip the dura
from the base of the skull, its free edge should be held
with some absorbent material, such as gauze, and
traction exerted.

   Any blood should be rinsed off the surface of the
brain with normal saline.   After a preliminary examination to note any conspicuous external abnormalities,
and any of the specimens referred to on p.1 have been
taken, the brain should be immediately suspended in
fixative.   If it is allowed to lie for even 10 to 15
minutes on the dissection bench, the brain becomes distorted;   and when it is dissected after fixation it is
not possible to assess herniation and shift accurately
as a result of post-mortem distortion of the ventricular
system.   Furthermore, such distortion prevents the
specimen being used as a source of illustrations for
publications or for teaching.

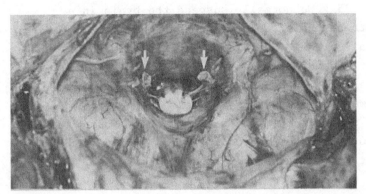

1.31

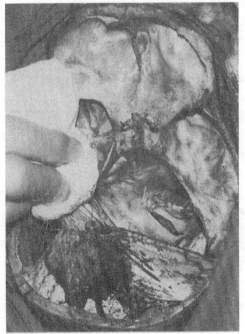

1.32

Figs. 1.33 - 1.35   We normally suspend the brain in a
10 litre polythene bucket about three quarters filled
with 10% formal saline.   We find a paper clip with one
end opened out a simple and satisfactory hook on which
to suspend the brain.   Once the brain has been almost
completely immersed in the fixative, the open end of the
paper clip is slipped under the basilar artery, care
being taken not to damage the pons.   When suspended the.
brain must not be in contact with the sides or the
bottom of the bucket since this will also cause distortion of the cerebral hemispheres.   It must also be
completely immersed.   The fixative should be changed
after 3 days and then at weekly intervals.   When the
fixative is being changed, the brain should be detached
from the paper clip to ensure that the basilar artery
does not tear, thus leading to problems in resuspending
the brain.

The major exception to immediate fixation of the
brain is the presence of subarachnoid haemorrhage
suggestive of a ruptured aneurysm on one of the arteries
at the base of the brain, since it is almost impossible
to dissect off fixed blood without damaging the arteries
or the aneurysm.   In these circumstances the arteries
at the base of the brain, including the middle cerebral
arteries in the Sylvian fissures and the anterior
communicating artery (common sites for aneurysms)
should be carefully exposed and blood clot washed off
with saline in an attempt to identify an aneurysm
before fixing the brain .

Brains should be fixed for 3 to 4 weeks prior to
dissection.

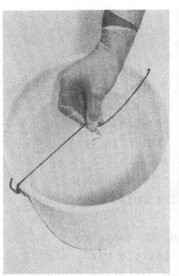

1.33

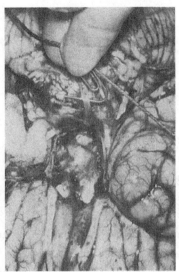

1.34

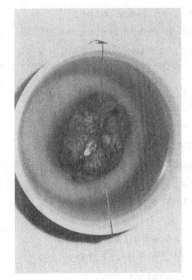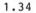

1.35

2.   The Base of the Skull

The base of the skull and its main anatomical
features are illustrated in Fig. 2.1.   The principal
structures that may require to be examined are the
pituitary gland, the cavernous sinuses, the trigeminal
ganglia and the middle ear.   The orbital contents are
considered separately in chapter 3.

The technique to be adopted depends on the circumstances of each individual case.   Thus the pituitary
gland is usually simply removed from the pituitary fossa
as shown in Figs. 2.2 - 2.6:   in a patient with an
adenoma of the pituitary gland, however, or some other
tumour that affects this region such as a chordoma, a
central segment of the base of the skull should be removed so that the extent of the tumour can be assessed,
e.g. to what extent an adenoma of the pituitary gland
has invaded into the cavernous sinuses or the adjacent
bone.   A similar technique should be used in a patient
suspected of having thrombosis of a cavernous sinus.
The block of bone removed can be decalcified, and
sections cut in the sagittal, horizontal or coronal
plane depending on the type of lesion that is being
investigated.

Using an electric saw with a fan-shaped blade, cuts
should be made along the lines indicated in Fig. 2.1:
this central block of bone can then be levered away
from the base of the skull after cutting through the
soft tissue in the nasopharynx.

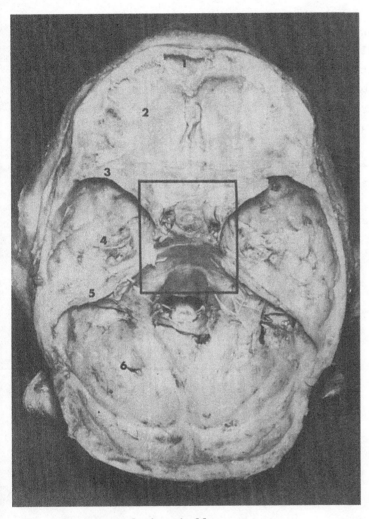

2.1   The base of the skull

    1. Frontal sinus
    2. Anterior cranial fossa (roof of orbit)
    3. Lesser wing of sphenoid bone
    4. Middle cranial fossa
    5. Petrous part of temporal bone to which
        tentorium cerebelli is attached
    6. Posterior cranial fossa

Fig. 2.2   The first step in removing the pituitary
gland is to incise the posterior margin of the
diaphragma sellae with a scalpel, the cutting edge of
the blade pointing upwards.   If this incision is not
made, the posterior lobe of the pituitary gland is almost invariably damaged when the posterior part of the
pituitary fossa is removed.

Figs. 2.3 and 2.4   Remove the posterior wall of the
pituitary fossa with a chisel (as shown here) or with
bone cutters.   This exposes the posterior surface of
the gland and an intact slightly protruding posterior
lobe (arrow).

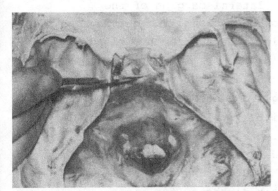

2.2

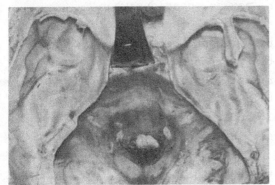

2.3

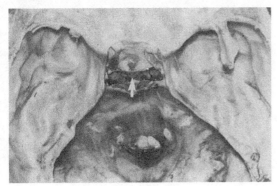

2.4

Fig. 2.5   The anterior and lateral margins of the
diaphragma sellae should now be incised, the cutting
edge of the blade again pointing away from the gland.

Fig. 2.6   The diaphragma should now be held with fine
forceps and the pituitary gland gently dissected free
from the pituitary fossa with a scalpel, the cutting
edge of the blade being directed towards the bone so
that no damage is inflicted on the pituitary gland.

        The pituitary gland should be fixed for at least
24 hours before it is further dissected for histological examination.   There may be occasions when a
sagittal section is indicated but in general the
greatest amount of information is obtained from a
horizontal block incorporating the anterior and the
posterior lobes.   This horizontal cut should be made at
the junction of the upper third and the lower two-thirds
of the gland.   Step serial sections may have to be cut
from the larger block in case any abnormalities are
restricted to its inferior portion.   The upper block
can either be examined in the horizontal plane or it can
be further dissected to obtain sagittal sections of the
lower part of the pituitary stalk.

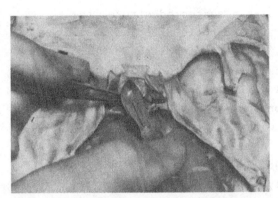

2.5

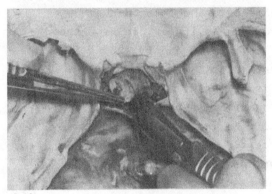

2.6

Fig. 2.7   In any patient with a suspected stroke, the
cavernous parts of the internal carotid arteries should
be examined as well as the neck arteries (see Chapter 5).
Once the pituitary gland has been removed it is very easy
to dissect off the lateral wall of the cavernous sinus
(held in this figure by forceps) to expose the internal
carotid artery (white arrow).

Fig. 2.8   The internal carotid artery enters the
cavernous sinus posteriorly from the carotid canal and
then arches anteriorly before turning upwards to enter
the subarachnoid space adjacent to the optic nerve.
The ophthalmic artery (arrow) takes its origin from the
internal carotid artery at this level and to expose it,
the anterior clinoid process (black arrow in Fig. 2.7)
has to be removed.   This is an essential step in
attempting to identify an aneurysm in this region.   In
this figure the upper end of the internal carotid artery
is being held with the forceps.

     Once exposed, the cavernous part of the internal
carotid artery may be transected in situ or cut into
serial transverse sections after removing it from the
cavernous sinus.

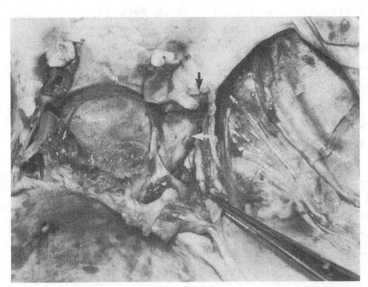

2.7

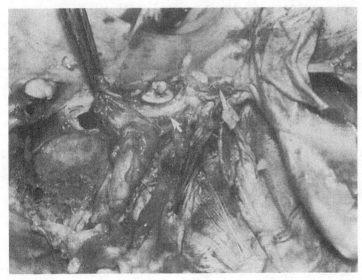

2.8

Fig. 2.9   The trigeminal ganglion lies in Meckel's
diverticulum on the superior surface of the greater wing
of the sphenoid bone.   To expose it (arrow) the dura
covering it has to be dissected from it.   The ganglion
can then be removed from the base of the skull.

Figs. 2.10 and 2.11   The only really satisfactory way
to examine the structures of the middle and inner ear is
to remove the large wedge of temporal bone as indicated
in the figure.   This block of bone must then be decalcified and large serial sections cut.   This,
however, is a specialised and time-consuming process
that is virtually only pursued by pathologists with a
special interest in otology.   It is, however, always
advisable to open the middle ears to ascertain if any
infectious process is present.   This can be done by
splitting the petrous part of the temporal bone with
a bone chisel as illustrated.

43

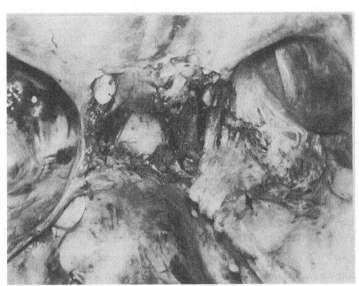

2.9

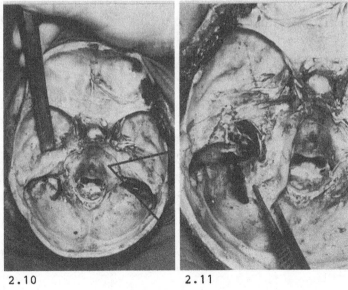

2.10   2.11

3.   The Eye and Orbital Contents

The eye should be removed at autopsy in neurological disorders involving the eye and brain (e.g.
multiple sclerosis, neuronal storage disorders and
temporal arteritis), in systemic disease with associated
ocular abnormalities (e.g. diabetes mellitus, hyper-
tension and leukaemia) and in primary disorders which
are of interest to ophthalmologists (e.g. previous
surgical intervention, glaucoma surgery, lens extraction,
degenerative diseases of the macula, optic atrophy etc.).
Removal of the eye itself will be dealt with before
a description of the exploration and removal of the
orbital contents is provided.

Fig. 3.1   Separate the eyelids with a self-retaining
retractor.

Fig. 3.2   With sharp pointed scissors separate the
conjunctiva from the sclera in a complete circle some
5-10 mm from the corneoscleral junction (the limbus).

Fig. 3.3   By traction on the conjunctiva free the
tissue from the sclera with sharp curved scissors.

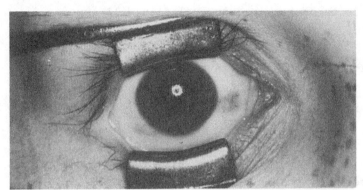

3.1

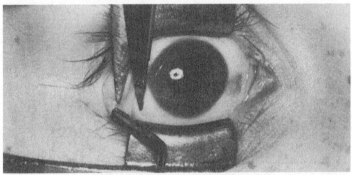

3.2

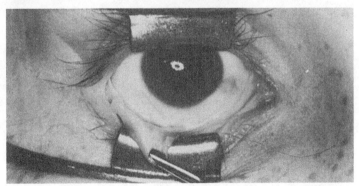

3.3

Fig. 3.4   Traction on the conjunctival flap will expose
the insertion of the medial rectus muscle (arrow).

Fig. 3.5   Insert a muscle hook into the orbit above the
medial rectus muscle, pass the hook behind the muscle
and pull the eye laterally.

Fig. 3.6   Dissect the soft tissue from the medial
rectus muscle (arrow) and divide the belly some 10-15 mm
behind the insertion.   This muscle will be used for
traction on the globe when the optic nerve is divided
(see Fig. 3.10).

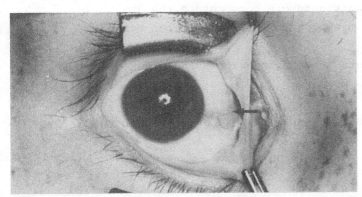

3.4

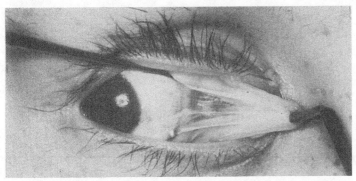

3.5

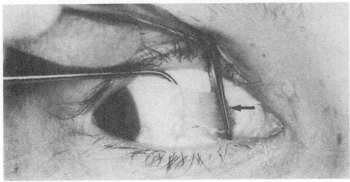

3.6

Fig. 3.7   Using the muscle hook rotate the eye
inferiorly and transect the superior rectus muscle.

Fig. 3.8   Rotate the eye superiorly and transect the
inferior rectus muscle.

Fig. 3.9   Rotate the eye medially and transect the
lateral rectus muscle.

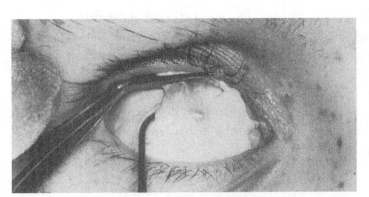

3.7

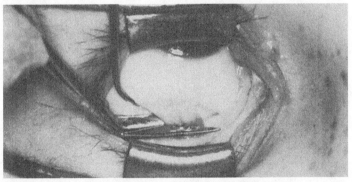

3.8

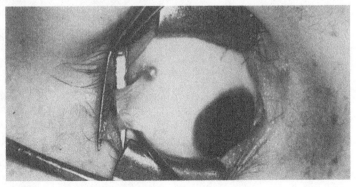

3.9

Figs. 3.10 and 3.11   Locate the medial rectus muscle
with fine forceps and then clamp the muscle with artery
forceps so that the eye can be pulled forwards (Fig.
3.11).

Fig. 3.12   Insert straight scissors along the medial
wall of the orbit and transect the optic nerve as far
posteriorly as possible.

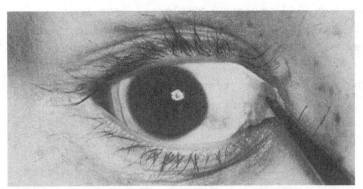

3.10

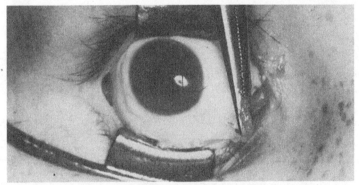

3.11

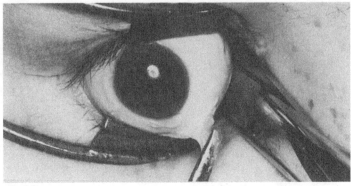

3.12

Fig. 3.13   The eye will prolapse completely from the
orbit.   The superior and inferior oblique (arrow)
muscles can now be transected.

Fig. 3.14   The remaining soft tissue can be cut through
and the eye with as large a portion of the optic nerve
(arrow) as possible removed from the orbit.

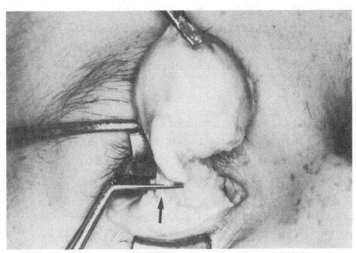

3.13

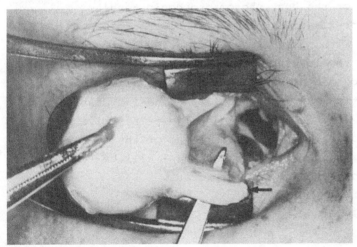

3.14

Fig. 3.15   Cotton wool is packed into the orbit leaving
sufficient space for an artificial eye.   If a prosthesis is unavailable, the insides of the lids may be
sutured to close the lids without any external
distortion.

Fig. 3.16   An artificial eye is inserted and the
residual conjunctival tissue is replaced in front of the
prosthesis.   The eyelids are partially closed and may
be fixed by sutures inside the lids.

   The enucleated eye may be fixed by immersion in
formal saline or in buffered glutaraldehyde (2.5%).
The former causes rapid opacification of the lens and
vitreous, and for the best photomacroscopic results
washing and post-fixation in 70% alcohol are to be
recommended.   With glutaraldehyde fixation a closer
resemblance to the in vivo appearance is retained and
the tissue is better preserved for electron microscopy.
Prolonged fixation may lead to collapse and indentation
in some eyes: if this occurs, injection of fixative
into the vitreous will restore the shape of the globe,
and after this further fixation the shape will be
maintained through the embedding process.

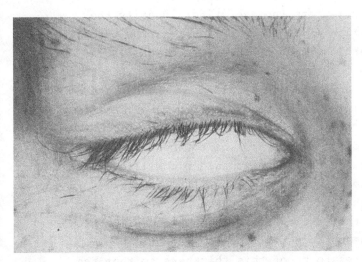

3.15

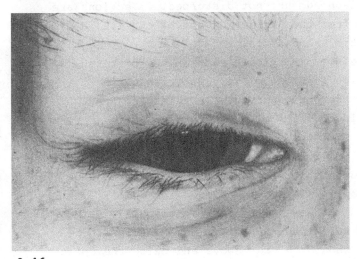

3.16

Fig. 3.17   To orientate the eye, first identify the
tendinous insertion of superior oblique (narrow arrow)
and the muscular insertion of inferior oblique (broad
arrow).   Since both muscles pass medially in the orbit
the top, the lateral and medial sides of the eye can now
easily be identified, and the eye correctly orientated
and located.   The long ciliary arteries run horizontally and if a cut is made parallel to these vessels it
will produce an accurate "horizontal" block (Fig. 3.18)
in which the macula will be in line with the disc.   In
conventional ophthalmic pathology the block taken from
the central part of the eye is between 5 and 8 mm thick
and includes the optic nerve, the lens and the pupil.
The block requires to be of this thickness so that the
lens and iris diaphragm are not disturbed.   Sections are
taken 3 to 4 mm from the surface of the block, i.e. as
near to its centre as possible.

Alternatively, a "vertical" section may be taken
at right angles to the long ciliary arteries on the
lateral side of the optic nerve.   In this case the
macula will be in the lateral or temporal calotte (cap)
of the eye.

Fig. 3.18   A horizontal section through an eye to show
the macula (arrow).   This cut was made for demon-
tration purposes to show the centres of the optic nerve
and the lens.   For histopathological examination the
horizontal cuts should be made above and below the optic
nerve in line with the edge of the cornea.

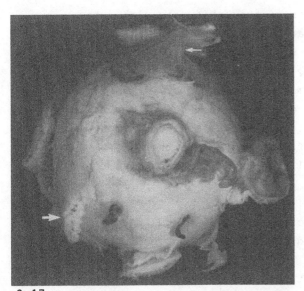

3.17

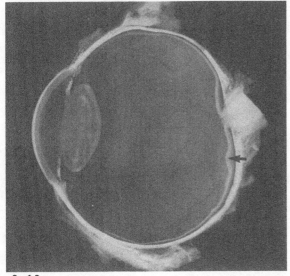

3.18

The entire contents of the orbit (the globe, the optic nerve, extraocular muscles, the lacrimal gland and orbital fat) should be removed in certain systemic (e.g. endocrine exophthalmos, giant cell arteritis etc.) or local diseases (inflammation, tumour etc.). They are best removed by exposure through the roof of the orbit. This dissection is easier if the tissues in the anterior part of the orbit are freed first since there is then less risk of cosmetically unacceptable damage to the eyelids.

Fig. 3.19   The conjunctiva is divided and freed from the sclera with pointed scissors as described on p.44.

Fig. 3.20   The supporting tissue around the anterior part of the eye is divided to the bony wall of the orbit.   It should now be possible to push the eye gently backwards into the orbit.   Any residual attachments to the lids should now be freed.

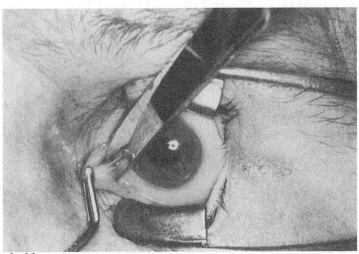

3.19

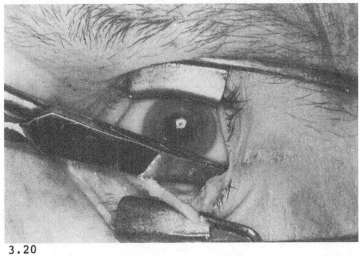

3.20

Figs. 3.21 - 3.23   After stripping the dura from the
base of the skull as indicated in Fig. 1.32, cut through
the roof of the orbit with an electric saw, preferably
with a fan-shaped blade, taking care not to damage the
optic nerve (arrow).

Fig. 3.24   Lift the bone flap off and remove any
residual bone with bone forceps.

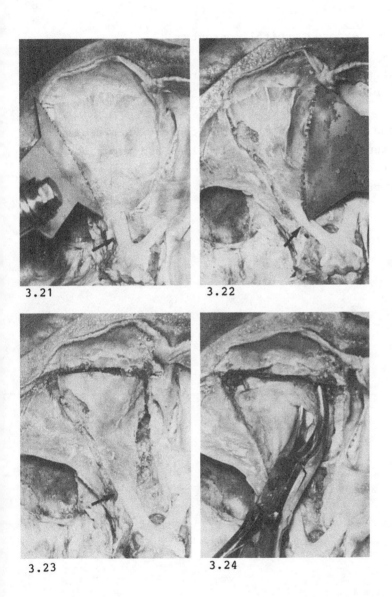

3.21

3.22

3.23

3.24

Fig. 3.25   The exposed orbital contents.

Fig. 3.26   Free the orbital tissues from the wall of
the orbit by blunt dissection using a spatula and forceps.

Figs. 3.27 and 3.28   Divide the firm connective tissue
ring around the optic nerve with a scalpel and separate
the orbital tissue from the wall of the orbit back to
the inferior orbital fissure (arrow).

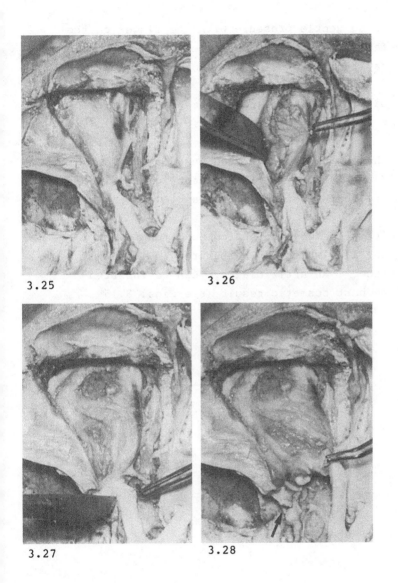

3.25

3.26

3.27

3.28

Fig. 3.29   Using gentle pressure with the finger on the anterior surface of the eye, push the eye backwards into the cranial cavity.

Fig. 3.30   Divide the inferior attachments of the eye and remove it from the orbit.

Fig. 3.31   The eye and the attached muscles and fatty tissue should be fixed in formal saline or glutaral- dehyde prior to further dissection (see p.54).

The orbit is packed with cotton wool to prevent collapse of the lids which can be sutured from the internal surface.   An artificial eye can be inserted to provide the best cosmetic result (see Figs. 3.15 and 3.16).

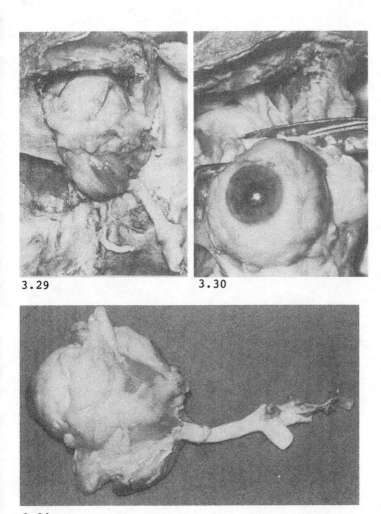

3.29   3.30

3.31

4.   The Spinal Cord

The spinal cord should be examined routinely in
every post-mortem examination on a patient with a disorder of the central nervous system.   This may, on
occasion, appear to be an unnecessary labour but even in
a patient thought to have died as a result of a severe
head injury, removal of the spinal cord may disclose
that there has been an unsuspected fracture/dislocation
of the cervical spine;   and in a patient known to have
a malignant brain tumour, examination of the spinal cord
may disclose that diffuse tumour or seedlings in the
spinal subarachnoid space have materially contributed to
the clinical picture.   And there are numerous metabolic
derangements including disseminated systemic malignant
disease where long tract degeneration in the spinal cord,
particularly in the posterior columns, has been the
principal source of neurological dysfunction.   If the
cord is not removed precise clinico-pathological
correlations can never be established in such cases.
    There is inevitably a certain reluctance on the
part of the pathologist and the mortuary attendant to
remove the cord because of the extra time and labour
involved.   In cases of particular interest, the best
technique is to remove the entire vertebral column so
that a careful dissection can be undertaken after
appropriate preliminary fixation but, using the anterior
approach illustrated here, removal of the spinal cord
and posterior root ganglia can with experience be
accomplished in little more than 10-15 minutes.   The

posterior approach (much used in the past) when the body
had to be turned over and a new skin incision made is
more time-consuming and less satisfactory for dissecting
out posterior root ganglia.   To make the removal as
easy as possible the ribs have to be cut through antero-
laterally to facilitate access of the saw to the
thoracic vertebrae, and the collar neck incision
illustrated in Fig. 5.1 adopted.   The vertebral column
should be extended by placing the head block under the
shoulders.

    Illustrating the precise technique has proved to be
very difficult, but this account should clarify the
basic principles.   Expertise will only be achieved by
practice.

Fig. 4.1   The basic principle in the anterior approach
to the spinal cord is to cut through the pedicles of the
vertebrae so that the cord can be exposed by removing
the vertebral bodies.   It can be seen from the figure
that the angle of the saw cut varies in different
regions of the vertebral column.   Thus in the lumbar
spine (a) the saw cut is almost horizontal;   in the
thoracic region (b) it is more oblique;   while in the
cervical region (c) it is almost vertical.

Fig. 4.2   An essential preliminary step in removing the
spinal cord is to free the dura around the foramen
magnum since it is very difficult to do this from below
when the spinal cord is finally being delivered.   Thus
after the brain has been removed, the dura adjacent to
the upper part of the spinal cord should be held with
toothed forceps and a scalpel inserted between the dura
and the vertebrae.   The dura should be freed around the
entire circumference of the cord, and it is usually
possible to achieve this over a distance of 2-3 cms.

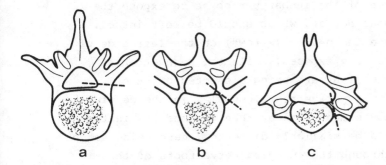

4.1

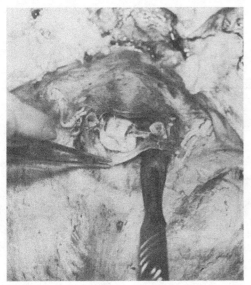

4.2

Fig. 4.3   The paravertebral muscles should be
dissected free of the lumbar vertebrae to expose the
emerging lumbar nerves, which should be left intact.
In this figure the nerves (arrows) on the left side of
the body have been exposed, while the paravertebral
muscles on the right are being dissected off the
vertebrae.   The paravertebral muscles in the cervical
region, although much smaller than the muscles in the
pelvis, should be similarly dissected, care being taken
not to cut through the emerging nerve roots of the
cervical plexus.

Fig. 4.4   The line of the saw cut in the thoracic
region should be cleared by incising the parietal
pleura (arrows) in the thorax immediately lateral to the
rib tubercules which can be easily palpated.

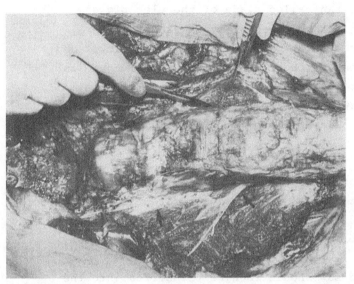

4.3

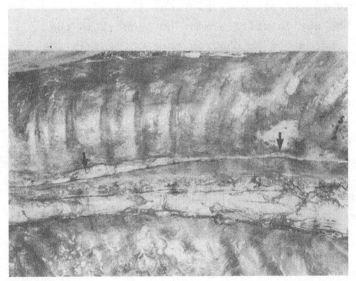

4.4

Fig. 4.5   The fan-tailed blade of the electric saw
should then be placed immediately in front of the
lumbar nerve roots (arrow) in the mid-lumbar level and
the pedicles cut through.   With the body flat on its
back, this cut is in the horizontal plane (see Fig.
4.1).   The saw will be felt to 'give' when the blade
enters the spinal canal, and it should not be allowed
to plunge.

Fig. 4.6   Continue sawing - again individual pedicles
will be felt to 'give' - in a caudal direction.   Once
the pedicle of the 5th lumbar vertebra has been cut,
make a deep oblique incision into the sacrum (arrow).

Fig. 4.7   The saw should then be reinserted into the
cut made in the mid-lumbar region, and the cut continued rostrally in the plane of section already
delineated.   The cut is still almost horizontal in the
lower thoracic region but it becomes more oblique in the
upper thoracic region.   If the angle and position are
correct, each individual pedicle will be felt to 'give'.
If this does not occur, the saw cut is not in the correct
plane.   In the cervical region (see Fig. 4.1), the saw
blade will be almost vertical in position, and at the
junction between the thoracic and cervical vertebrae
(arrow) the angle of sawing changes quite abruptly.
The cut should be continued rostrally to the base of the
skull, care being taken in the cervical region not to
allow the saw blade to plunge through the cervical
nerve roots.
     A precisely similar sequence of steps has now to
be undertaken on the other side.   When the oblique cut
is made this time in the sacrum, a large wedge of the
sacrum will be felt to spring free.
     If there is some deformity of the vertebrae, e.g.

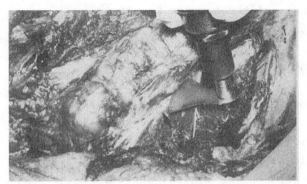

4.5

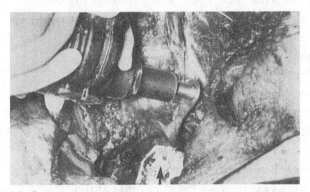

4.6

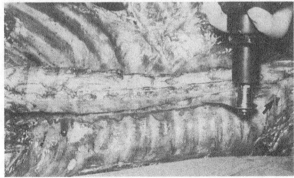

4.7

kyphoscoliosis, the angle of the saw cut has to be
adapted to the position of the pedicles.

Figs. 4.8 and 4.9   The next stage is to lift the
vertebral bodies from the canal thus exposing the
anterior surface of the spinal cord (arrow).   This is
not difficult provided that the saw cuts have been in the
proper plane.   Starting in the lumbo-sacral region, the
vertebral bodies should be pulled forward and any
adhesions between the dura on the ventral surface of the
cord and the vertebral bodies cut with a scalpel (Fig.
4.9).   This process should be continued rostrally until
the lumbar, thoracic and cervical vertebral bodies can
be retracted in a single block.

Fig. 4.10   The entire length of the spinal cord is now
exposed, and if the sawing has been done properly, the
dura should be intact.   This should always be the aim
because it means that there will have been no direct
damage to the cord, and that it will not become distorted in the course of fixation.   This illustration
shows the lower thoracic and lumbar regions and the
lumbar nerve roots.

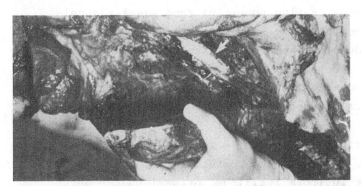

4.8

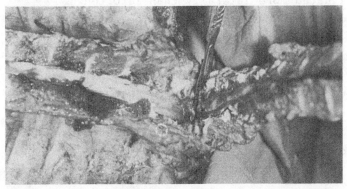

4.9

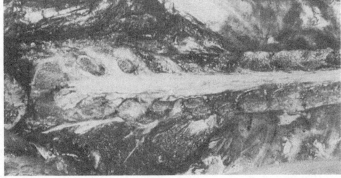

4.10

Fig. 4.11   Representative posterior root ganglia should
always be removed with the spinal cord.   If the
previous procedure has been undertaken correctly it is
very easy to dissect out lumbar (arrows) and sacral
posterior root ganglia and the proximal parts of the
lumbar and sacral nerves.

Fig. 4.12   Further dissection is required in the
cervical region to expose the posterior root ganglia.
These are large fusiform swellings (arrows) on the nerve
roots and are situated more laterally than is often
thought.   The cervical nerve roots should be followed
from the spinal cord and the bone adjacent to the inter-
vertebral foramina dissected away to expose the ganglia.
This dissection should be continued to the proximal
part of the nerve distal to the ganglion.   With this
exposure it is remarkably easy to dissect out the
entire brachial plexus if there is any indication for
subjecting it to histological examination.

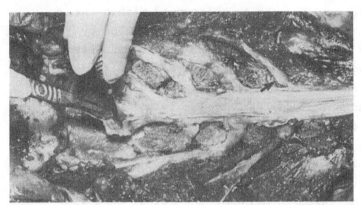

4.11

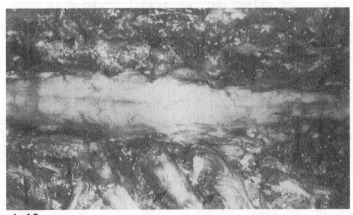

4.12

Fig. 4.13   The cord has now to be removed within the
dura.   This is probably most easily accomplished by
placing artery forceps (arrow) on the lumbar dura without compressing any of the nerve roots deep to it.   The
lumbar and sacral nerves are then transected distal to
the ganglia and the caudal part of the spinal cord
lifted from the vertebral canal.   There are always
some adhesions between the dura and the vertebral arches
and these should be cut with a scalpel.

    This procedure should be continued rostrally,
great care being taken to maintain the spinal cord as
straight as possible since any sharp angulation will
produce post-mortem structural damage.   If the cervical
cord at the foramen magnum has been freed as indicated
on p. 68, the entire spinal cord with attached nerve
roots and root ganglia will slide free of the vertebral
canal.

Fig. 4.14   In patients where the principal lesion is
thought clinically to be affecting the caudal brain stem
and/or the upper cervical segments of the spinal cord,
the latter have to be removed still attached to the
brain.   To achieve this, a wedge of occipital bone and
the arches of the upper three or four cervical vertebrae
have to be removed.   A mid-line incision is made in the
skin covering the occipital bone and the upper cervical
region, and the skin reflected.   The dura should now be
separated from the occipital bone using a spatula as
indicated in Fig. 1.10 before making an oblique saw cut
(arrows) in the occipital bone from the edge of the
original saw cut in the skull to the foramen magnum.

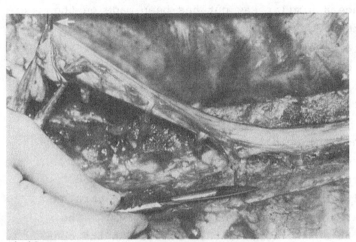

4.13

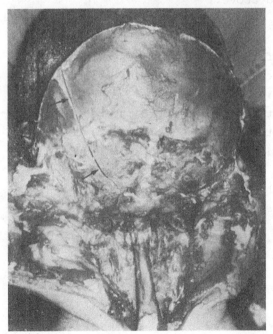

4.14

Fig. 4.15   Once a similar saw cut has been made on the
other side, the wedge of occipital bone is removed to
expose the dura covering the cerebellum.   The next step
is to dissect off the posterior paravertebral muscles so
that a saw cut (arrows) can be made through the laminae
of the upper cervical vertebrae.

Fig. 4.16   Once the spinal cord has been transected,
the cervical segments can be freed from the vertebral
canal.   Before removing the brain with the attached
upper cervical segments of the spinal cord, the dura has
to be opened at the level of the foramen magnum.   The
remainder of the spinal cord is then removed in the conventional manner described above.

    Once the spinal cord has been removed, the vertebral
canal should be examined for any abnormalities such as
disc protrusions, extradural spinal tumour, or evidence
of a fracture or dislocation.
    If the dura is intact, the spinal cord may be fixed
in the bucket along with the brain.   If, however, the
dura has been opened, it is advisable to open the dura
over the entire length of the spinal cord anteriorly and
posteriorly, and to fix the spinal cord suspended in a
large measuring cylinder so that no distortion occurs
during fixation.

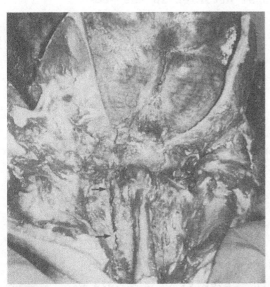

4.15

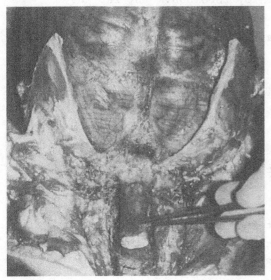

4.16

5.   The Extracranial Cerebral Arteries in the Neck

No post mortem examination on a patient who has
died as a result of a stroke, or who has a history of
a previous stroke, is complete unless the major extracranial cerebral arteries, viz. the internal carotid
and the vertebral arteries in the neck, are examined
since cerebral infarction may be caused or contributed
to by occlusion or stenosis of one of these arteries.
They can be opened in situ but this does not really
allow of an assessment of the severity of stenosis or
the extent of any occlusion by thrombus.   By far the
best method is to dissect out the principal arteries
and then to examine them after preliminary fixation.
This dissection should be undertaken before removing
the central structures of the neck, viz. the pharynx,
larynx etc.

Fig. 5.1   Access to the arteries is greatly
facilitated by using a "collar" incision when opening
the body, and then reflecting the skin to expose the
lateral structures in the neck.

Figs. 5.2 and 5.3   The sternomastoid muscle (arrow in
Fig. 5.2) is retracted laterally to expose the common
carotid artery (arrow in Fig. 5.3).

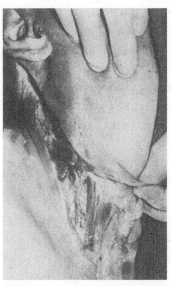

5.1

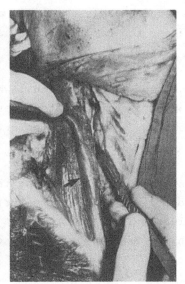

5.2

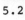

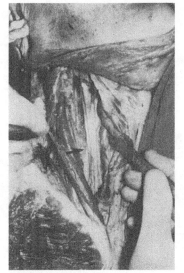

5.3

Fig. 5.4   Continue the dissection in an upwards
direction to clear the carotid arteries rostral to the
carotid sinus (arrow).

Fig. 5.5   Continue the dissection downwards to expose
the bifurcation of the innominate artery (thick arrow)
and then dissect out the subclavian artery (narrow
arrow).

Fig. 5.6   Continue dissecting along the subclavian
artery to expose the origin of the vertebral artery
(arrow) and clear this to the point at which it enters
the foramen in the transverse process of the sixth
cervical vertebra.

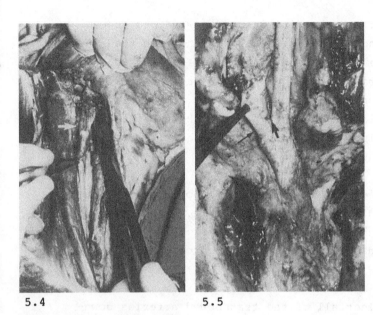

5.4

5.5

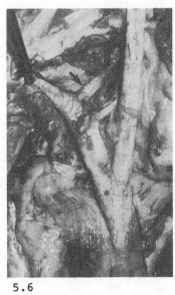

5.6

Fig. 5.7 Continue the dissection downwards to expose
the arch of the aorta (thick arrow), and then the
origins of the left common carotid and subclavian
arteries (narrow arrows), the latter arising from the
arch of the aorta distal to the former.   Now dissect
out the arteries on the left side of the neck to expose
the carotid sinus and the origin of the left vertebral
artery from the subclavian artery.

Fig. 5.8 All of the major arteries should now be transected as high in the neck as possible.   In this
figure the right internal and external carotid arteries
are being transected distal to the carotid sinus
(arrow).

Fig. 5.9 Reflect all of the transected arteries downwards to the arch of the aorta.

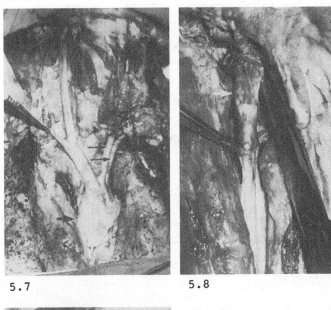

5.7

5.8

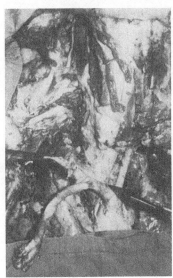

5.9

Figs. 5.10 and 5.11 The final stage is to cut a wedge
from the arch of the aorta incorporating the origins of
the major neck arteries.   Serial transverse cuts -
preferably after fixation - can now be made along all of
the arteries to assess the presence of stenosis and/or
occlusion.   The arteries should not be completely
transected so allowing preservation of the specimen
until, if indicated, representative blocks are taken for
histological examination.

　　　1.   Arch of aorta
　　　2.   Innominate artery
　　　3.   Common carotid arteries
　　　4.   Subclavian arteries
　　　5.   Origins of vertebral arteries
　　　6.   Carotid sinuses

　　There are occasions on which the vertebral arteries
require to be examined in detail.   They can be dissected out of the transverse processes of the cervical
vertebrae at the time of autopsy but it is often pre-
ferable to remove the cervical vertebrae and the bone
adjacent to the foramen magnum in one block.   This can
then be fixed and decalcified before dissecting out the
arteries, or making serial horizontal sections.

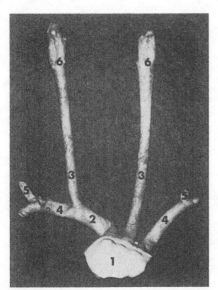

5.10

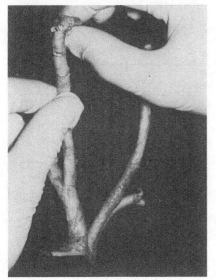

5.11

6.   Muscle and Nerve

Widespread sampling of peripheral nerve and muscle
is essential in any patient thought to have had some
type of neuromuscular disease.   Many of the enzyme
histochemical techniques routinely used in the examination of muscle biopsies can still be applied to
muscle taken up to 24 to 36 hours after death.   Thus
some specimens of muscle taken post mortem should -
properly labelled - be frozen in liquid nitrogen as
quickly as possible.   Most specimens of nerve and
muscle are, however, simply fixed in neutral 10% formal
saline.   The selection of muscles and peripheral
nerves to be examined will be determined by the clinical
pattern of the disease, and prior discussion with the
appropriate clinician is therefore essential.   For a
complete picture of peripheral neuropathy, cranial
nerves, the trigeminal ganglia, posterior root ganglia
and various peripheral nerves need to be examined.
Once the posterior root ganglia in the lumbar and sacral
region have been exposed (see Figs. 4.11 and 4.12) it is
not difficult to continue the dissection distally to
free all of the major nerves constituting the brachial
plexus.   Other nerves can be sampled individually.

This is a rather expert field, however, and before
undertaking a post-mortem examination on a patient known
to have some disorder of muscle or peripheral nerve it
is advisable also to consult a neuropathologist.   It
may, for example, be important to attempt to examine

the small muscles of the hand, and intramuscular nerves
and end plates adjacent to the motor point in a muscle.

Fig. 6.1   The muscle to be sampled should be widely
exposed - in this illustration, the triceps brachii.
Since precise longitudinal and cross sections will be
required in subsequent histological studies, the piece
of muscle removed should as far as possible be along
the line of the fibres.   For a large muscle, remove a
strip some 3 by 1.5 by 1.0 cm.

Fig. 6.2   It is important to ensure that the muscle
does not become distorted in the course of fixation.   A
simple method of achieving this is to place the strip of
muscle slightly stretched on a piece of firm card to
which the name and side of the muscle can be applied.
If this is left exposed to the air for 5 or 10 minutes
the muscle will not become detached from the card when
it is placed in fixative.   After preliminary fixation,
longitudinal and transverse blocks can then be easily
obtained.

    More than one sample of muscle can be placed on the
same card.

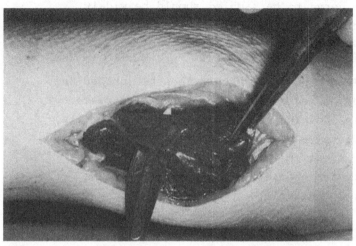

6.1

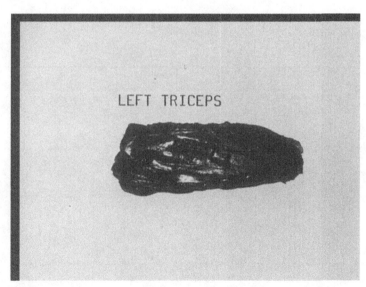

6.2

Fig. 6.3   The nerve to be sampled should be widely
exposed, in this illustration the median nerve in the
forearm (arrows).

Fig. 6.4   A length of nerve should then be removed and,
as with muscle, placed slightly stretched on a piece of
firm card.   In addition to the name of the nerve, its
proximal and distal ends should be clearly labelled.
Once again the specimen should be left exposed to air
for 5 to 10 minutes before it is placed in fixative.
(P = proximal, D = distal).

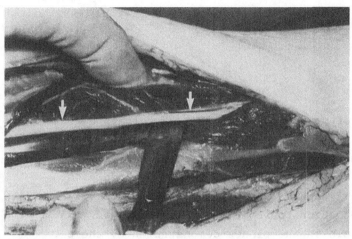

6.3

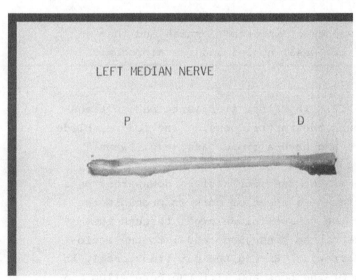

LEFT MEDIAN NERVE

P   D

6.4

7.   Dissection of the Fixed Brain

The type of dissection depends to a certain extent
on the site of any abnormality suspected of being
present.   Thus if there is thought to be a midline
lesion affecting the third or the fourth ventricle, a
midline sagittal section may be indicated (Figs. 7.23 -
7.25) and on occasion there may be good reason for
slicing the brain in the planes demonstrated by the C-T
head scanner.   In general, however, the method
described below is the most informative since it pro-
duces the maximum amount of information about distortion
of the brain, the size and shape of the ventricular
system, the presence of internal herniae and the
appearances of the basal nuclei and the hippocampus
(Ammon's horn).

Figs. 7.1 and 7.2   The first step is to make a transverse cut through the rostral pons.   The scalpel blade
should be large and have a broad base (e.g. Swann-
Morton No. 22).
Place the brain, superior surface downwards, on a
non-slippy surface - a sheet of cork is probably the
best.   Insert the scalpel blade right through the
lateral surface of the pons just caudal to the oculomotor nerves (arrow).   Extend the cut transversely to
the other side of the pons and lift the cerebellum and
the brain stem away from the cerebral hemispheres.
Care must be taken not to damage the medial parts of
the temporal lobes with the scalpel.

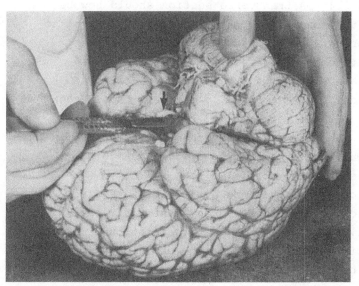

7.1

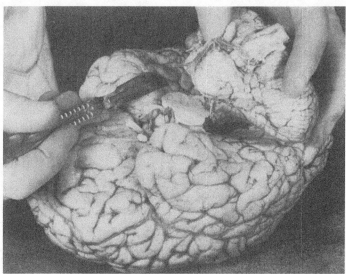

7.2

Figs. 7.3 and 7.4   A transverse section should now be
made through the rostral midbrain immediately rostral to
the oculomotor nerves (arrow).   This is one of the
more difficult cuts and the scalpel should be pushed
through the lateral part of the midbrain parallel to
the previous cut.   The transverse incision should then
be continued to the other side and the midbrain
detached from the cerebral hemispheres.   Particular
attention should again be paid to avoiding damaging the
temporal lobes with the scalpel.

A block of midbrain is now available if required
for histological examination and any tentorial
herniation, i.e. medial and downward herniation of the
medial part of the temporal lobe (the parahippocampal
gyrus), will be clearly seen.

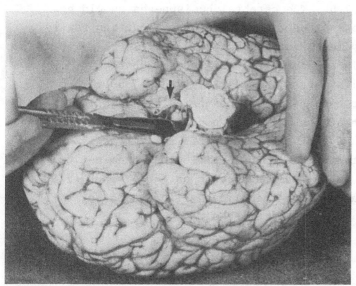

7.3

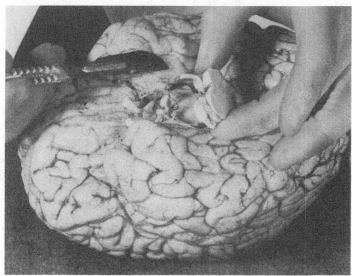

7.4

Figs. 7.5 and 7.6   The cerebral hemispheres should now
be cut into coronal sections.   The first cut can really
be made at any level but a relatively easy level at
which to obtain a symmetrical cut is through the
mamillary bodies (arrow), preferably at the junction of
their anterior two-thirds and posterior one-third.
This ensures that the mamillary bodies are seen in the
brain slices and that there is sufficient tissue in the
anteriorly situated block for histological examination.
The first cut is of the greatest importance, since if it
is asymmetrical, all of the slices will also be so.

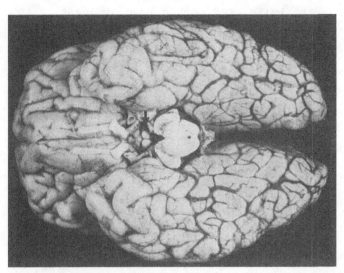

7.5

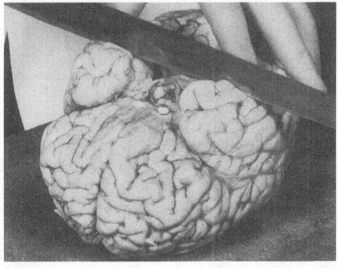

7.6

Figs. 7.7 and 7.8   The knife used should have at least
a 10" blade, preferably thin rather than thick but as
rigid as possible, and should of course be sharp so that
there is no need for a sawing action.   The first
coronal section should be made in one long, smooth cut.

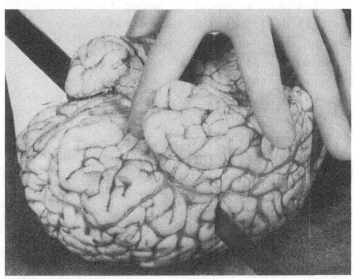

7.7

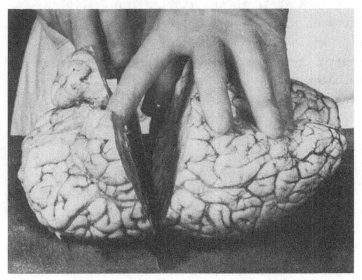

7.8

Figs. 7.9 - 7.11   The next stage is to obtain coronal
slices of the cerebral hemispheres of an even and known
thickness so that the antero-posterior extent of any
lesion identified can be measured.   A very simple
technique is to use two metal bars of an appropriate
size and shape placed on a cork mat so that they do not
slip.   The cutting angles illustrated in Fig. 7.9 are
made of 1 cm square brass.   The longer arm of the angle
measures 17 cm and the shorter arm 14 cm.   Considerable
downward pressure has to be exerted on the brain to
prevent it rising up, since if this occurs the slice is
inevitably of varying thickness.   It is also important
to angle the knife slightly downwards so that it remains
in close contact with the cutting angles.   If this is
not done, the knife tends to lift off the angles again
producing a slice of uneven thickness.   The pathologist
should cut away from himself to the midline (Fig. 7.10)
and then back towards himself to complete the cut (Fig.
7.11).   A sawing action should be avoided but this is
sometimes necessary if the knife encounters a tough
tumour, or a haematoma.

    It is of course possible to cut slices less than
1 cm thick by using thinner cutting angles.

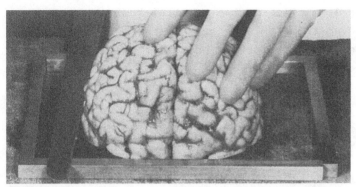

7.9

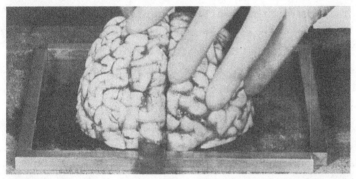

7.10

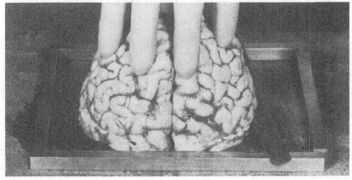

7.11

Fig. 7.12   The 1 cm slice of the cerebral hemisphere
can now be removed from the cork mat and further 1 cm
slices made from the anterior and posterior parts of
the cerebral hemispheres.

Figs. 7.13 and 7.14   It is advantageous to change the
angle of the cut in the occipital lobes so that the
knife cuts through the calcarine sulcus (arrow) at
right angles.   A further 1 cm thick slice can then be
obtained from the occipital poles.
      The oblique cut means that there is one rather
thick section of brain in the posterior parietal region
which measures 1 cm wide inferiorly but up to 3 cm wide
superiorly.   If, therefore, there is any lesion in the
posterior parietal or occipital regions whose size
should be measured, conventional coronal sections
should be continued to the occipital poles.
      In laying out the slices for examination, a system
should be adopted whereby either the anterior or the
posterior surface of each slice faces upwards.   This
is simply a matter of preference but it is important to
be consistent so that there is never any problem in
differentiating the left from the right hemisphere,
either when demonstrating the brain or when examining
photographs of the specimen.

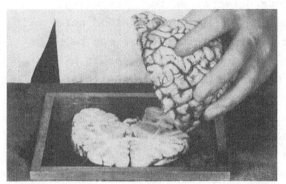

7.12

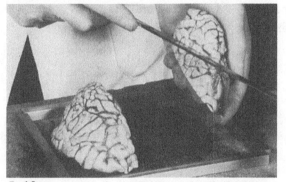

7.13

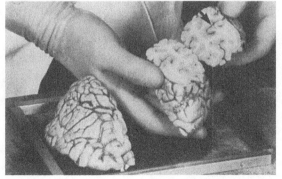

7.14

There is no one standard technique for dissecting
the brain stem and cerebellum.   The one described here
is in many ways the most informative but there may be
occasions when the brain stem and cerebellum should be
dissected in one block, usually in the horizontal plane.

Figs. 7.15 - 7.17   Separate the brain stem from the
cerebellum with a scalpel or a brain knife.   In Fig.
7.15 a cut is being made through the left middle
cerebellar peduncle with the knife angled slightly to
the pons, and the cut is then continued to the lateral
part of the fourth ventricle.   A similar cut is then
made on the other side and the brain stem detached
from the cerebellum.

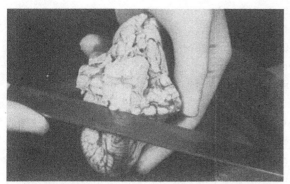

7.15

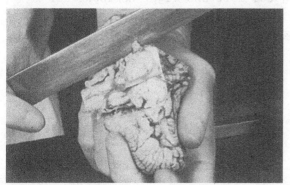

7.16

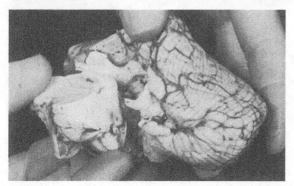

7.17

Figs. 7.18 - 7.20   Each cerebellar hemisphere should
be cut at right angles to the folia.   The first cut
should be made at the junction between the medial third
and the lateral two-thirds of the hemisphere since this
will cut through the dentate nucleus (arrow in Fig.
7.19).

Slices 1 cm thick (Fig. 7.20) can then be cut from
each hemisphere of the cerebellum.   Again consistency
must be maintained in laying out the slices for
examination and demonstration so that there is no
possibility of confusing the left and right hemispheres.

A final cut should be made in the mid-line through
the vermis of the cerebellum.

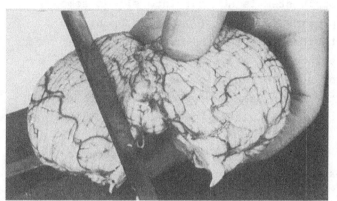

7.18

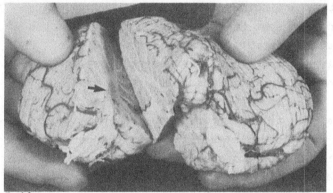

7.19

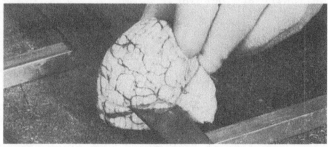

7.20

Fig. 7.21   The brain stem is now cut into slices some
2-3 mm thick to provide sections of midbrain, pons and
medulla.   As with the slices of the cerebral hemispheres and the cerebellum, a system has to be adopted
whereby either the superior or inferior surfaces of
each segment of the brain stem always faces upwards so
that left and right can be clearly defined.

Fig. 7.22   This illustration shows a brain dissected by
the technique described on the preceding page.   The
pathologist will more often than not be aware of abnormalities in the brain in the course of obtaining the
conventional slices, and he may decide that it would be
advantageous to obtain some thinner slices if he suspects
that a lesion, e.g. a stereotactic pallidotomy or
thalamotomy, is likely to be small.   Nevertheless, the
full extent of any abnormality is rarely appreciated
until the entire brain is examined.   It is not our
intention in this book to illustrate pathology but it is
useful to recall that in unilateral lesions, the contra-
lateral hemisphere is a useful control in assessing the
extent of abnormalities in the affected hemisphere, and
in sections laid out as depicted here it is very easy to
identify distortion, shift and herniae.

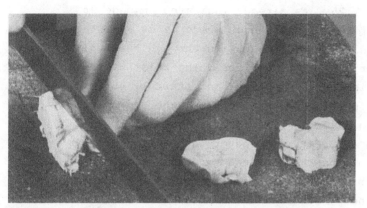

7.21

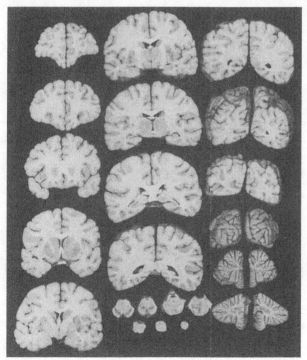

7.22

Figs. 7.23 - 7.25   As already indicated on page 96
there are certain circumstances where it is advantageous
to make a midline sagittal section through the brain.
There are various techniques for doing this but probably
the easiest is to use a scalpel and start by cutting
through the rostral end (the genu) of the corpus
callosum (Fig. 7.23).   This cut can then be continued
rostrally to the posterior end of the corpus callosum
(the splenium) and then through the midline of the
brain stem, bisecting the basilar artery on the ventral
surface of the pons.

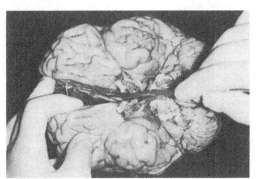

7.23

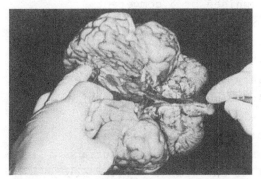

7.24

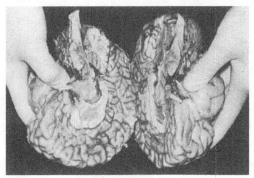

7.25

8.   The Anatomy of the Brain

As indicated in the preface, this chapter is not intended to be a detailed atlas of neuroanatomy.   Its aim is simply to illustrate the principal anatomical structures in the brain, using photographs rather than diagrams, that should be recognised by a competent pathologist, if only to allow him to state reasonably precisely the site of any lesion identified post mortem. Provided slices of uniform thickness have been cut as described on p.104 using a very simple technique, the pathologist will also be able to measure the size of any abnormality with a reasonable degree of accuracy.

The first four illustrations demonstrate the principal structures on the medial and lateral surfaces of the brain and at the base of the brain.   These are followed by a series of coronal slices of the cerebral hemispheres.   Fig. 8.11 includes the mamillary bodies and represents the first cut made in the cerebral hemi- spheres as suggested on p.100.   Thus Figs. 8.5 to 8.10 are anterior to this first cut, and Figs. 8.12 to 8.20 behind it.   With the aim of illustrating as many levels as possible, Figs. 8.11 to 8.17 have been cut at 5 mm intervals using angles 5 mm thick but similar in all other respects to those illustrated in Fig. 7.9.   We have attempted as far as possible to restrict key numbers to one hemisphere so that the corresponding structure in the other hemisphere can be clearly seen. Finally, there are illustrations of the cerebellum and the brain stem obtained as shown in Figs. 7.18 to 7.21.

The cerebellum is a rather complex anatomical structure
and only major anatomical structures are labelled.

Many structures appear on more than one photograph
and they are therefore not always labelled so as to
reduce the numbers on individual photographs.

It does not matter if it is the anterior or the
posterior surfaces of the slices of cerebral hemispheres
that face upwards, or the superior or inferior surfaces
of the slices of the brain stem. What does matter is
consistency so that the pathologist when examining the
slices - or particularly photographs of the slices -
knows immediately which is the left side, and which is
the right. The ensuing illustrations depict the
posterior surface of each slice of cerebral hemisphere,
the medial surface of each slice of cerebellum, and the
superior surface of each slice of brain stem. A
similar system should be adopted when taking blocks for
histology: thus we always cut the surfaces illustrated
so that the pathologist will always be able to dis-
tinguish left from right provided that there are one or
more distinctive anatomical features, e.g. Ammon's horn
or basal nuclei, in the block. If there is none, he
must be careful to label blocks left or right. A
technique sometimes adopted is to make a small wedge-
shaped notch, or even a hole with a miniature type cork
borer, in the blocks taken from one side of the brain.

Figs. 8.1 and 8.2   The lateral and medial surfaces of
the brain

1. Superior frontal gyrus
2. Middle frontal gyrus
3. Inferior frontal gyrus
4. Sylvian fissure
5. Superior temporal gyrus
6. Middle temporal gyrus
7. Inferior temporal gyrus
8. Precentral gyrus
9. Central sulcus
10. Post central gyrus
11. Superior parietal lobule
12. Inferior parietal lobule
13. Lateral occipital gyri
14. Paracentral lobule (parietal lobe)
15. Cingulate gyrus
16. Medial occipital (including calcarine) cortex
17. Corpus callosum - genu
18. Corous callosum - body
19. Corpus callosum - splenium
20. Anterior commissure
21. Posterior commissure
22. Pineal gland
23. Lateral ventricle
24. Third ventricle
25. Aqueduct
26. Colliculii
27. Fourth ventricle
28. Cerebellum
29. Mid-brain
30. Pons
31. Medulla

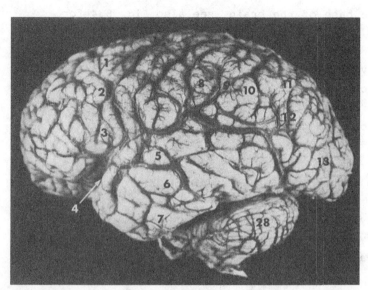

8.1

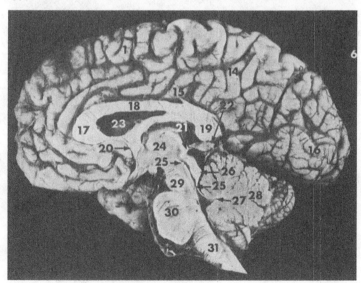

8.2

Fig. 8.3   The base of the brain (see also Fig. 8.4 for more detail).

1.   Olfactory bulb
2.   Gyrus rectus
3.   Medial orbital gyri
4.   Lateral orbital gyri
5.   Temporal pole
6.   Uncus
7.   Fusiform gyrus
8.   Inferior temporal gyrus
9.   Pituitary stalk and median eminence
10. Mamillary body
11. Basilar artery
12. Pons
13. Medulla
14. Cerebellar hemisphere
15. Cerebellar tonsil

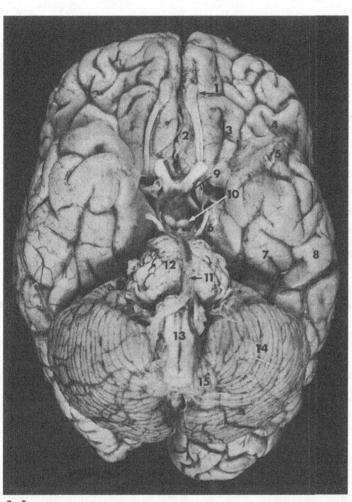

8.3

Fig. 8.4   The central part of the base of the brain
(same brain as illustrated in Fig. 8.3).

1. Olfactory tract
2. Anterior communicating artery
3. Optic nerve and chiasma
4. Upper end of internal carotid artery
5. Middle cerebral artery entering Sylvian fissure
6. Anterior choroidal artery
7. Posterior communicating artery
8. Oculomotor (third cranial) nerve
9. Origin of posterior cerebral artery partly
    obscured by oculomotor nerve
10. Trigeminal (fifth cranial) nerve
11. Sixth cranial nerve
12. Facial (seventh cranial) and auditory (eighth
    cranial) nerves
13. Vertebral artery (this degree of asymmetry is not
    uncommon)
14. Posterior inferior cerebellar artery
15. Origins of lower cranial nerves
16. Pyramid

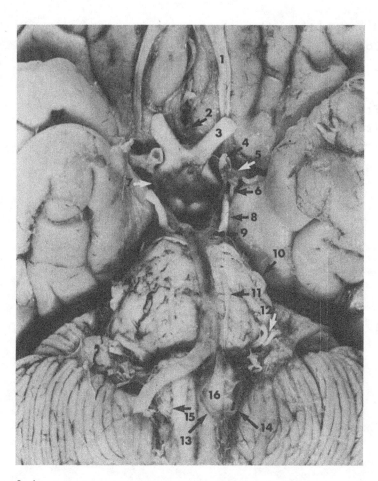

8.4

Figs. 8.5 and 8.6   Slices through the anterior part of
the frontal lobes.

1.   Superior frontal gyrus
2.   Superior frontal sulcus
3.   Middle frontal gyrus
4.   Middle frontal sulcus
5.   Inferior frontal gyrus
6.   Orbital gyri - medial and lateral
7.   Gyrus rectus

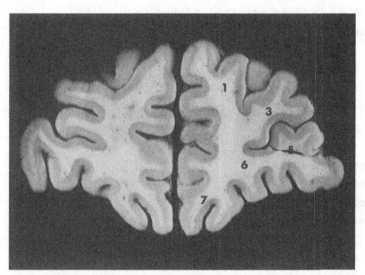

8.5

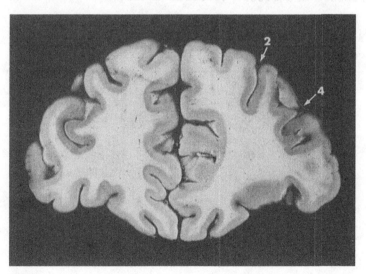

8.6

Figs. 8.7 and 8.8   Slices at level of the genu of the
corpus callosum.

1.   Superior frontal gyrus
2.   Superior frontal sulcus
3.   Middle frontal gyrus
4.   Middle frontal sulcus
5.   Inferior frontal gyrus
6.   Orbital gyri - medial and lateral
7.   Gyrus rectus
8.   Cingulate gyrus
9.   Genu of corpus callosum
10. Anterior horn of lateral ventricle
11. Anterior cerebral artery
12. Pericallosal artery
13. Sylvian fissure and middle cerebral artery
14. Temporal pole
15. Olfactory tract
16. Head of caudate nucleus
17. Putamen

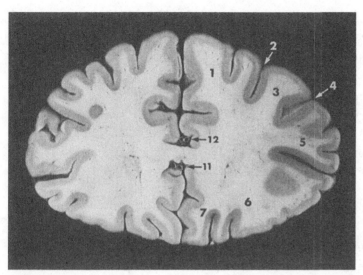

8.7

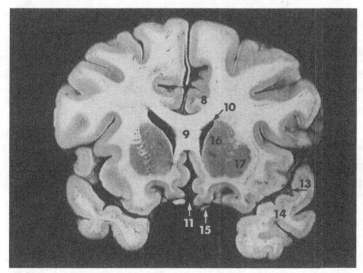

8.8

Figs. 8.9 and 8.10   Slices at level of the anterior
basal ganglia.

1. Superior frontal gyrus
2. Superior frontal sulcus
3. Middle frontal gyrus
4. Middle frontal sulcus
5. Inferior frontal gyrus
6. Cingulate gyrus
7. Sylvian fissure
8. Insula
9. Superior temporal gyrus
10. Superior temporal sulcus
11. Middle temporal gyrus
12. Middle temporal sulcus
13. Inferior temporal gyrus
14. Inferior temporal sulcus
15. Fusiform gyrus
16. Uncus
17. Corpus callosum
18. Pericallosal artery
19. Caudate nucleus
20. Internal capsule
21. Putamen
22. Globus pallidus
23. Claustrum
24. Amygdaloid nucleus
25. Anterior commissure
26. Optic chiasma
27. Optic tract
28. Interventricular septum
29. Interhemispheric fissure

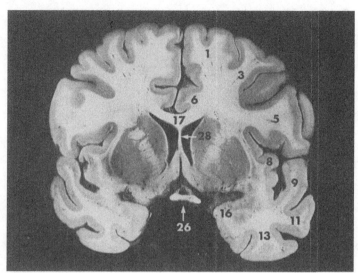

8.9

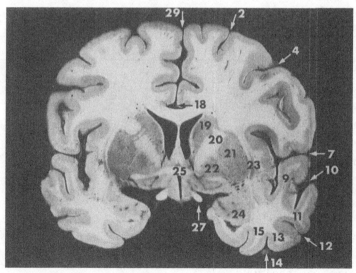

8.10

Figs. 8.11 and 8.12   Slices through the posterior part
of the hypothalamus

1. Cingulate gyrus
2. Superior frontal gyrus
3. Superior frontal sulcus
4. Middle frontal gyrus
5. Middle frontal sulcus
6. Inferior frontal gyrus
7. Insula
8. Superior temporal gyrus
9. Superior temporal sulcus
10. Middle temporal gyrus
11. Middle temporal sulcus
12. Inferior temporal gyrus
13. Inferior temporal sulcus
14. Fusiform gyrus
15. Collateral sulcus
16. Parahippocampal gyrus
17. Ammon's horn (hippocampus)
18. Corpus callosum
19. Body of lateral ventricle
20. Interventricular foramen (Monro)
21. Third ventricle
22. Mamillary body
23. Caudate nucleus
24. Internal capsule
25. Putamen
26. Globus pallidus
27. Optic tract
28. Fornix
29. Anterior part of thalamus
30. Cerebral peduncle

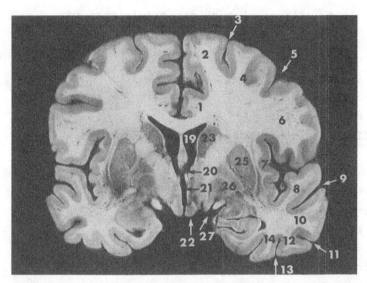

8.11

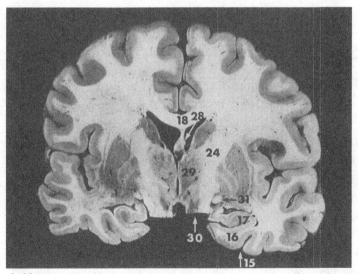

8.12

Figs. 8.13 and 8.14   Slices through the middle part of
the thalamus.

1. Interhemispheric fissure
2. Precentral gyrus
3. Middle frontal gyrus
4. Inferior frontal gyrus
5. Sylvian fissure with branches of middle cerebral
    artery
6. Insula
7. Superior temporal gyrus
8. Middle temporal gyrus
9. Inferior temporal gyrus
10. Fusiform gyrus
11. Parahippocampal gyrus
12. Ammon's horn (hippocampus)
13. Caudate nucleus
14. Putamen
15. Globus pallidus
16. Internal capsule
17. Thalamus - anterior nucleus
18. Thalamus - medial nucleus
19. Thalamus - lateral nuclear complex
20. Thalamus - dorsolateral nucleus
21. Subthalamic nucleus
22. Lateral ventricle and interventricular septum
23. Interventricular foramen of Monro
24. Third ventricle
25. Red nucleus
26. Substantia nigra
27. Posterior cerebral artery
28. Cerebral peduncle

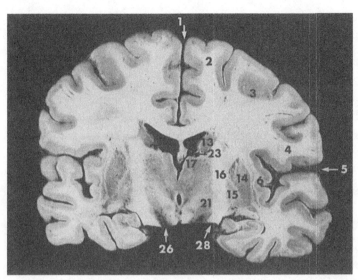

8.13

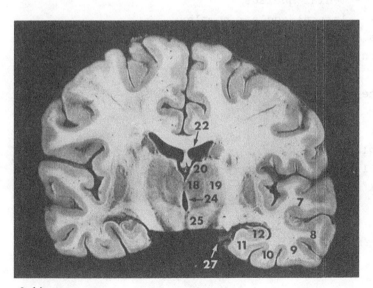

8.14

Figs. 8.15 and 8.16   Slices through the posterior part
of the thalamus.

1.   Precentral gyrus
2.   Postcentral gyrus
3.   Inferior frontal gyrus
4.   Sylvian fissure
5.   Insula with adjacent branches of middle cerebral
     artery
6.   Superior temporal gyrus
7.   Middle temporal gyrus
8.   Inferior temporal gyrus
9.   Fusiform gyrus
10. Parahippocampal gyrus
11. Hippocampus (Ammon's horn)
12. Lateral geniculate body
13. Thalamus - medial nucleus
14. Thalamus - lateral nuclear complex
15. Thalamus - pulvinar
16. Third ventricle
17. Fornix
18. Cingulate gyrus
19. Aqueduct
20. Superior colliculus
21. Pineal gland
22. Body of lateral ventricle
23. Temporal horn of ventricle

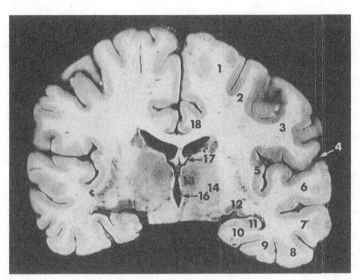

8.15

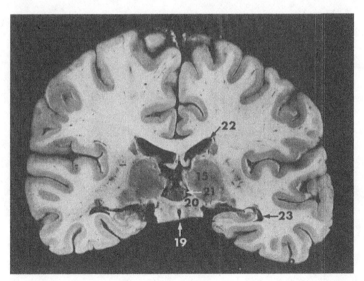

8.16

Figs. 8.17 and 8.18   Slices at level of the splenium
of the corpus callosum.

1.   Splenium of corpus callosum
2.   Superior parietal lobule
3.   Inferior parietal lobule
4.   Superior temporal gyrus
5.   Middle temporal gyrus
6.   Inferior temporal gyrus
7.   Fusiform gyrus
8.   Parahippocampal gyrus
9.   Ammon's horn (hippocampus)
10. Fornix
11. Cingulate gyrus
12. Thalamus - pulvinar
13. Posterior cerebral artery
14. Occipital horn of lateral ventricle
15. Paracentral lobule

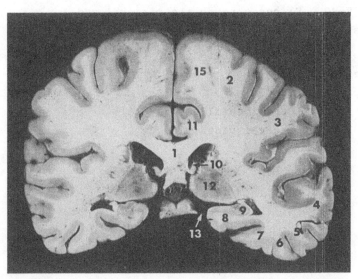

8.17

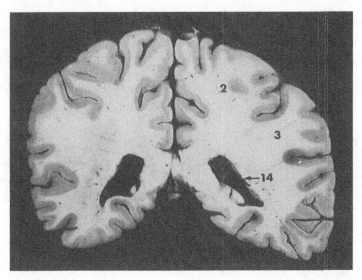

8.18

Figs. 8.19 and 8.20   Slices through the parietal and
occipital lobes.

1.   Superior parietal lobule
2.   Intraparietal sulcus
3.   Inferior parietal lobule
4.   Occipito-temporal gyri (medial and lateral)
5.   Occipital horn of lateral ventricle
6.   Calcarine sulcus
7.   Calcarine cortex

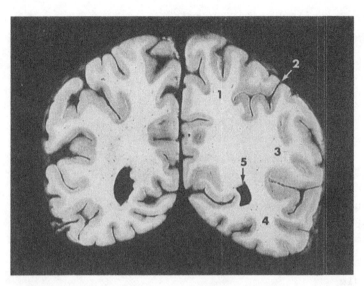

8.19

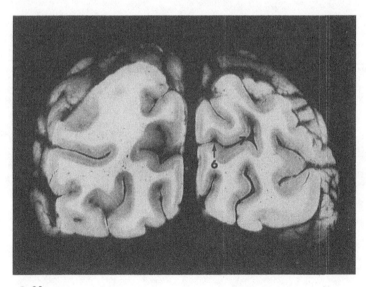

8.20

Fig. 8.21   The Cerebellum   (a)   vermis
                              (b)   medial third
                              (c)   lateral third

 1.   Culmen
 2.   Declive
 3.   Folium
 4.   Tuber
 5.   Pyramid
 6.   Uvula
 7.   Dentate nucleus
 8.   Middle cerebellar peduncle
 9.   Tonsil
10.   Superior surface
11.   Dorsal angle
12.   Inferior surface

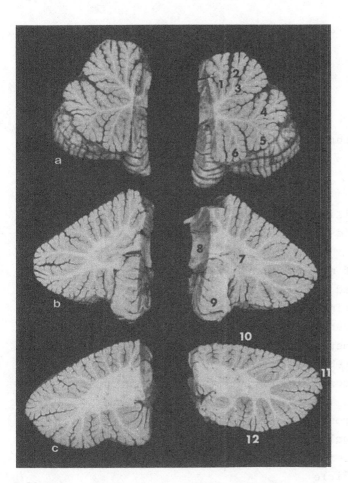

8.21

Fig. 8.22   The Brain Stem   (a)   mid-brain
                               (b)   rostral pons
                               (c)   mid-pons
                               (d)   rostral medulla
                               (e)   caudal medulla

Only gross structures are labelled since individual
nuclei can only be identified precisely in histological
sections.

1.   Inferior colliculus
2.   Tectum of mid-brain
3.   Aqueduct
4.   Tegmentum of mid-brain and pons
5.   Region of red nucleus
6.   Substantia nigra
7.   Cerebral peduncle
8.   Oculomotor nerve
9.   Superior cerebellar peduncle
10. Superior medullary velum
11. Basis pontis (incorporating nuclei pontis and
     descending cortico-spinal tracts)
12. Pigmented nucleus of pons (locus coeruleus)
13. Trigeminal nerve
14. Fourth ventricle
15. Middle cerebral peduncle
16. Inferior cerebellar peduncle
17. Region of hypoglossal and vagal nuclei
18. Inferior olivary nucleus
19. Pyramid
20. Gracile nucleus
21. Cuneate nucleus
22. Decussation of pyramidal tracts.

143

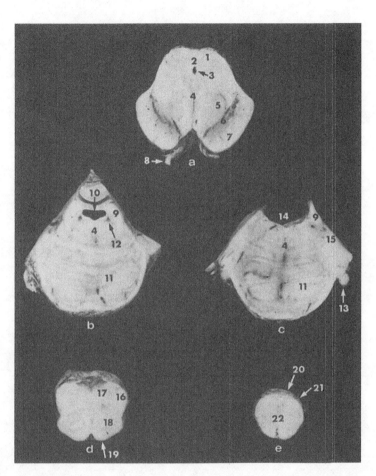

8.22